The Tiger Within

Practical Self Defense in a Modern World

How to bring out your INNER TIGER
when you need it most

By John Munro

Note

Physical conflict is inherently risky. The best way to deal with physical conflict is to take all reasonable steps to avoid it before it occurs. Even practicing responses to violence in a controlled environment is not without risk. Whenever practicing such responses, your own safety and that of your partner should be your first priority. Only ever practice at a speed and with a level of force that both you and your partner are comfortable with.

Inflicting bodily harm on another person is generally a crime unless there is a legal justification. The laws governing the infliction of bodily harm for self defense purposes vary by jurisdiction. You should familiarize yourself with the applicable laws governing the use of force for self defense in the jurisdiction you live in.

This book is for informational purposes. There is no guarantee that the use of the information contained in this book will be successful in preventing injury to yourself or those with you in any particular situation. The author and publisher are not liable for any damage or injury or other adverse outcome resulting from the application of information contained in this book.

ISBN 978-0-473-13714-4

Published by Infosource Ltd
Auckland
New Zealand

Cover design by John Munro
Cover design © 2008 John Munro

To George,
my little tiger

Table of Contents

Introduction

Have you ever seen a dog attack a cat?

What normally happens? That's right; the cat normally turns tail and is out of there like a streak, quickly getting to safety.

What about when the dog is too close, or the cat can't find anywhere to run?

Have you ever seen that cat turn and send the dog packing?

I have. Many times.

Usually it goes something like this. The cat has been walking along somewhere, minding its own business, when suddenly out of the blue a much larger, ferocious looking dog has run at the cat, barking and snapping its mouth.

The cat has turned towards the dog and in an instant arched its back, bristled its fur, made an angry face and hissed. Sometimes this has been enough for the dog to decide it is just not worth it and back off. If the dog has continued to approach or lunge, the cat has yowled and swiped its claws across the dog's nose and eyes several times in quick succession, its paws moving like a blur until the dog has retreated, usually emitting a very surprised yelp as it turns tail and runs the OTHER way.

Of course it doesn't always play out this way.

Sometimes the cat will freeze up, or react slowly and passively. If this is the case, the results aren't pretty.

So what is the difference between the cat that sends the dog packing, and the one that ends up falling victim to the dog's vicious attack?

Somewhere deep inside the first cat there was a TIGER lurking. A TIGER which the cat brought out when it was needed most.

Each of us is similar to the cats in this story. Over thousands of years we have become domesticated. Most of us no longer need to go out and hunt and kill for food to survive. We are also not compelled to fight predators on a regular basis to protect ourselves and our families. We have adapted to a modern environment with different demands on our bodies and minds. Our reactions are moderated to fit within our social environment.

For the most part this is great. We live longer, happier, more fulfilled lives as we are able to devote our energies to other pursuits, developing in the areas of art, technology, sports and so on.

However our society is becoming more violent. For more and more of us there will be instances in our lives when we are placed under threat of violence. Our normal daily reactions we have developed as a result of living in our modern societies are not suitable for dealing with these threats. If we continue to use these reactions at the time when we are under threat of violence we will tend to act slowly, passively or even freeze up, much like the second cat in our story.

Fortunately, just like the first cat, each of us also has a TIGER lurking deep within us. The innate ability to bring out our primitive reactions and transform into a fighting animal. An animal capable of acting and reacting to defend ourselves and our families when faced with a violent attack. Whether this Tiger comes out when it is needed depends on how well we have prepared ourselves mentally and physically.

This book will teach you how to prepare yourself so that your INNER TIGER will come out when you need it most.

How to use this book

Most of us have heard of the 80/20 rule. We get 80% of our results from the things that take only 20% of our time and effort. In a violent, unpredictable confrontation, 80% of the outcome will be determined not by how fit you are, how strong you are, or whether you are an accomplished martial artist, but by how well you have prepared yourself psychologically to deal with the situation.

All too often we get things reversed and spend 80% or more of our time on the activities that only bring 20% of the results. This can make the task seem daunting, as you have to work much, much harder to get the same end results. This book focuses on the "80%" component of self defense - your mental preparedness and strategies, so you will be ready to act when the time comes.

Chapter one of this book examines the physiological changes that occur when we are faced with a dangerous situation and how we can reinterpret them to our advantage.

Chapter two looks at how we can begin to move past ideas about violence that we have been pre-conditioned into, so that we can be most effective in defending ourselves.

Chapter three revisits the example of the cat with the INNER TIGER, identifying lessons we can learn from the example of this cat, both in terms of day to day preparation and also action when the time comes that it is needed. The following chapters then go on to apply those lessons to our daily lives and situations.

Chapters four through six look at how you can prepare so that you can relax in your environment and reduce the chances of actually experiencing a violent confrontation.

Chapters seven through ten cover practical information and strategies of how to physically deal with a violent confrontation should you need to.

The analogy of the INNER TIGER is used throughout.

It is recommended that you read this book through from start to finish completing the exercises you will encounter along the way. Then reread the book a second time completing the mental exercises again with the benefit of any additional knowledge you have gained through the process of reading the book. Many of the exercises are mental, requiring you to identify things in your environment or to imagine yourself in certain situations. The more you do these exercises the more skilled you will become at them. The imagined situations will become more realistic, and your mind will more quickly come up with solutions to them. This will carry over into more immediate physical actions when you need them.

You may find it helpful to review specific sections of this book several times until you have fully absorbed their contents, particularly chapters eight, nine and ten as they contain information about dealing with violent situations which may take several reviews to come to grips with.

Chapter ten contains examples of some common types of violent attacks and how you can deal with them. This chapter is designed to help you see how you can apply the principles discussed throughout the earlier sections of this book. It does not cover every possible situation, no book can. It WILL show you how the same simple principles can be applied to multiple situations, giving you the confidence to act using simple, natural and effective strategies without worrying about a 'right' technique for a particular scenario.

You will gain a lot simply from reading through chapter ten, but to gain the full benefit you will need to practice at least some of these applications with a partner. While mental preparation makes up the 80% that will primarily determine our effectiveness in a self defense situation, the remaining 20%, or physical experience, is still important. Doing at least some physical practice creates neural pathways that will help to turn your mental preparations into physical action when the time comes.

Practicing these scenarios and techniques will prepare you to use some of the most simple and effective methods to deal with an attacker. It will not however make you an expert in all possible self defense situations. If possible, it is recommended that you also attend classes with a qualified self defense instructor to gain further in depth instruction on how to use your body most effectively in a violent situation.

Chapter One: The moment of truth

This is the deciding moment, the moment that decides whether deep down we are a TIGER or just another domestic cat. This is the moment when we become aware of an existing or impending threat, and it is time for us to act.

Most likely this moment will come unexpectedly, when you are out for an evening having a good time, going about your daily business, or even relaxing at home. It may come in the form of criminals seeking material goods, a predator seeking sex or, as unfortunately is becoming more and more common, simply mindless violence.

Whatever form it takes there will be a moment in time when you become aware that you or your loved ones are under threat of physical violence. How you respond at this very moment will largely determine what follows - whether you successfully repel your attacker, or whether you become another victim. How you respond in this moment will be determined primarily by whether you have prepared yourself psychologically (mentally).

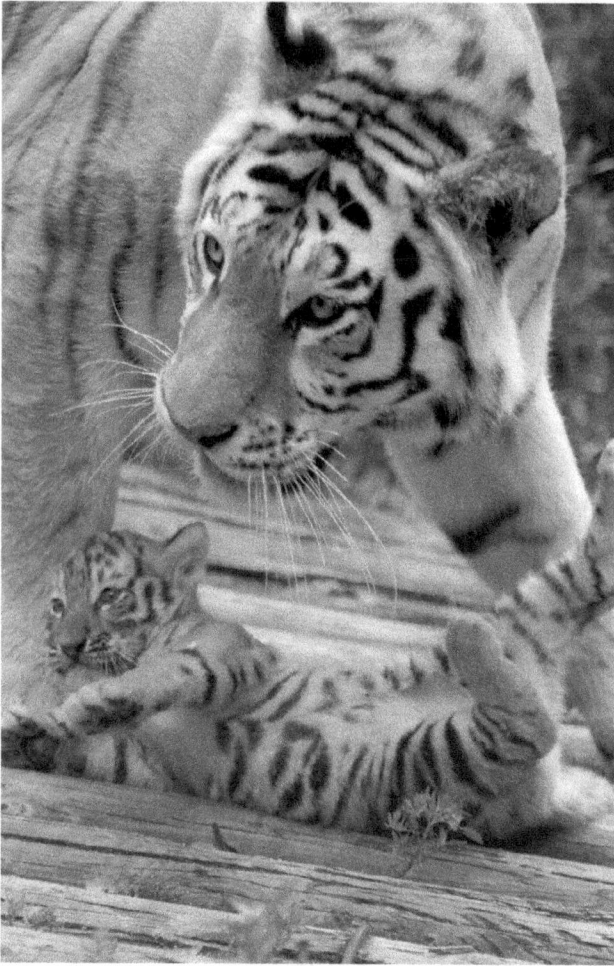

At this moment a number of physiological (bodily) changes occur. When we sense a threat, our bodies start to release large amounts of adrenalin into the bloodstream. Our pupils dilate our heart beat quickens, we breathe deeper, our hair may even stand on end (much like a cat's). The action of our digestive organs is inhibited, and blood and nutrient flow to our muscles increase. To put it simply, our body switches on, prepared to take sudden action.

At the same time activity in the front or logical part of our brain is reduced and activity in the lower rear part of the brain responsible for instinctive behavior increases. Our body prepares us to act naturally, pushing aside logic and reason so that our instincts will not be inhibited.

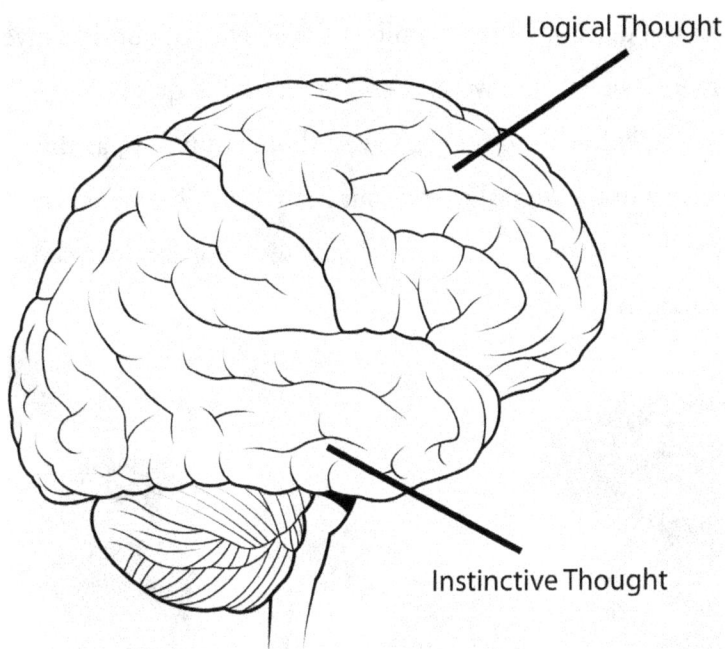

Logical Thought

Instinctive Thought

This state is commonly referred to as 'fight or flight.' It is interesting to note that our bodies undergo many of the same physiological changes when we are excited, angry or even just intensely interested.

Think of the young couple out on a date. Sitting across a candlelit table, the pupils dilate showing interest. The heart races as that special someone makes a move closer. Our breathing deepens. We might feel a little chill up and down our spine. We may even go off our food and not feel like eating as our body is sending so much energy to other parts of our body that it inhibits the activity of our digestive organs. In the end we may end up behaving quite illogically, much to the dismay of those around us, as the activity in the logical part of our brain is inhibited and the activity in the instinctive part increases. You see love can be dangerous too...

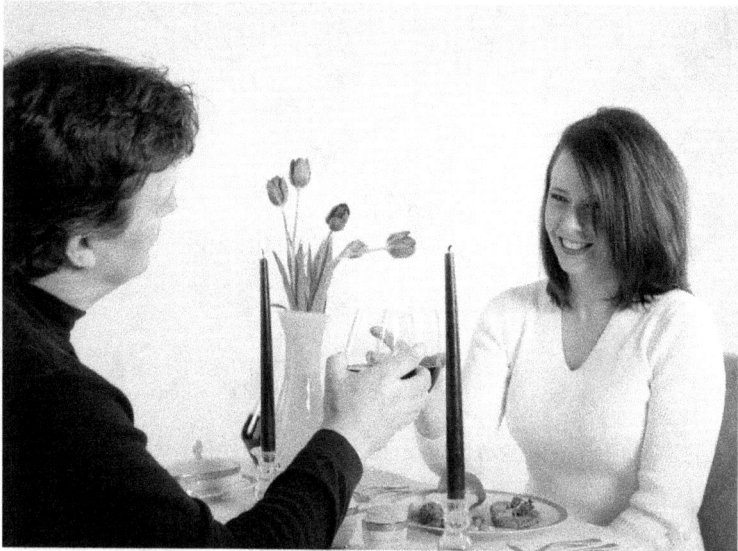

Think also of what happens when someone gets very angry. The eyes widen, the pulse races, breathing quickens, energy rushes to the muscles (people can perform feats of prodigious strength when they are angry enough), the activity in the logical part of the brain is reduced and instinctive behavior increases – resulting again in people sometimes doing things which are quite illogical but seemed quite natural to them at the time.

Researchers have actually shown that whether we interpret these changes in our bodies as fear, excitement or anger is largely determined by what we have conditioned ourselves to believe about the situation.

Now... I am not suggesting we need to fall in love with danger and violence, or develop an anger problem in order to be able to defend ourselves. The key is to remember that these changes are simply a natural and useful response of our body to the situation; we do not need to **interpret** them as fear.

Accept these changes and use them to your best advantage. You will feel a surge of energy. Your reactions will be faster, your strength greater. You will not perceive fine detail as clearly, but you will be able to sense things like movement more easily and respond faster. This is an excellent condition to be in should you have to either 'fight or take flight'.

The problem arises when the condition goes from 'fight or flight' and turns into 'freeze'. This occurs when either we are faced with a situation so far outside of our experience, real or imagined, that we do not have strong instinctive programming to deal with it, or when our instincts come up against strong programming which conflicts with our instinctive desire to protect ourselves (what could this programming be? See the next chapter). Remember our logical brain is inhibited, our instinctive brain takes over and will do the best it can with what it has programmed in there. If it's got no relevant programming, or the programming involves too great an internal conflict there is little it can do.

Either way, the result is inaction.

When the moment of truth comes it is time to act. If you are prepared, you WILL act when the time comes. Choose now to interpret the sensations you will feel, simply as your body switching on preparing to deal with the situation. Think of all you have to live for, your family, friends, and loved ones. Think of the things you still want to do in your life, the people you want to see, the places you want to go. Let this combine together into a fierce determination and will to live. This will help you to appreciate the sensations of your body switching on and interpret them in a way that will give you the confidence and resolve you need to act effectively.

You have taken the first step in your preparation by reading this book. By absorbing the information in this book and completing the exercises, you will be putting neural programming in place that will allow you to act quickly, decisively and in a way that is logical and effective. When the moment of truth comes, the time for thinking and planning has passed. By thinking out and practicing your actions before the moment of truth comes you will ensure that you act automatically and effectively, instead of possibly acting illogically, ineffectively, slowly, or worse freezing up and not acting at all.

Chapter Two: Shaking off domestication

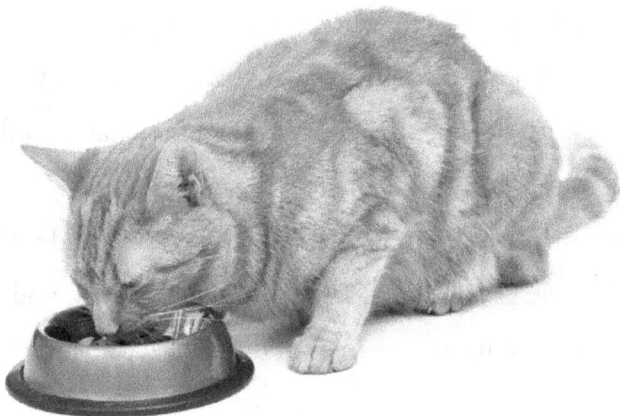

Right from when we are born, we are taught to be nice to others. We are told not to hit our brother when he pinches us. We are taught that we should share our toys. We are taught that the answer to just about everything is to be nice to each other and treat others with respect.

This is good. It enables us to spend extended periods of time in close proximity with others. It allows us to greet strangers without fear and welcome them into our circle of friends and acquaintances. It creates an environment where we can create relationships of trust and co-operate with one another. It underpins the functioning of our society on every level.

However there are some who choose to violate that trust, some that choose to act in a way that tears at the very fabric of our society. When this happens the rules change and it is back to the 'law of the jungle'. It can take some preparation for our minds to adapt to operating under this law when we have become so conditioned to living under the spoken and unspoken rules of our civilized society.

We can begin this preparation by considering the different situations and environments in which we might face an attack. This might be on the street, in the office, on the train, in the bedroom, in the kitchen etc.

Exercise 1:

Identify a situation where you may be attacked. Now play through in your mind what may occur. Make it as realistic as possible.

Picture an attacker. What direction might they come from? How do they attack? Do they grab at you? Do they strike with their hands or a weapon? What do you do? What are your options in this situation? Are there any weapons available to you? (more details on how you can deal with an attack and weapons of opportunity are found in later chapters of this book). See in your minds eye how you successfully fend off or escape your attacker. Then relax.

Some of you may find this exercise difficult. This is because your mind does not already have readily available to it information about how to deal with these situations. Don't worry too much about this. You will gain the information you need as you proceed through this book. Once you have read this book all the way to the end, come back and repeat the exercises again and notice the increased confidence you now have in dealing with this situation.

By running through the situation in your mind you are starting to put programming into the instinctive part of your brain that will allow you to deal with this situation or a similar one should it ever happen. When the time comes you will already have the programming in there and a number of available options which will allow your reactions to be faster and more confident in dealing with the situation.

Exercise 1 continued:

Now play through the same scenario again, this time engaging more of your senses and mentally putting yourself inside the situation. See out of your eyes in the situation, hear from your ears, smell from your nose and feel with your skin.

What are you wearing? What does it feel like on your skin? What can you smell? Air freshener? Perhaps you can smell your attackers sweat? What can you see as you look around? What can you hear? Is there music playing? Can you hear your own breathing? Feel yourself successfully fending off or escaping your attacker.

Now relax.

Check how you feel. If you feel tense at all, you can now imagine yourself going to a safe, enjoyable relaxing situation. Maybe in one of your favorite places. Maybe the beach, maybe somewhere you've been on holiday. Again engage your senses of sight, sound, touch, smell and even taste and just enjoy the experience relaxing in this new safe enjoyable situation. Check how you feel. Continue with this exercise until you feel completely relaxed and at ease.

Repeat this exercise using different methods of escaping your attacker, be creative. Also repeat for a number of different situations.

The more of our senses we engage, the more realistic we can make the scenario in our minds, the stronger the neural pathways we will form in our brains and the easier it will be for us to access and use them when the appropriate time comes. To some extent our brains can not really tell the difference between what we imagine and what we actually experience. Some researchers suggest that this is in fact what we are doing when we dream - coming up with likely scenarios and playing through actions that will help us to get through them. Our brains think the situations are so real that if we did not have a special little trick whereby our bodies are effectively paralyzed when we slip into a deep sleep, we would actually physically act out the scenarios. When we jump or kick in our sleep, we are on the very verge of falling into a deeper slumber and this handy mechanism has not yet kicked in. People who sleepwalk (or sleep whatever other activity you can imagine) have a problem where this mechanism does not engage properly all the time. By consciously creating and playing through some useful self defense scenarios, we are preparing our minds to set our bodies into appropriate action when required. Also by running through these scenarios and then relaxing afterwards we are preparing our bodies to let go of the stress easily should we ever experience an actual situation of this type.

The other thing we need to address at this stage is our concept of violence. Culturally we are conditioned to certain ideas about violence. We have see things on TV or movies, we may have seen kids fighting or guys getting into arguments in a bar, we may have seen professional or amateur fighters compete in sporting contests in a ring. Much of this fighting is what would be considered play fighting in the wild. Most of it is about dominance, proving who is tougher. While people may get hurt, it is largely about knocking the other person down, or causing the opponent to submit to our will. The 'claws' don't really come out in this kind of fighting.

This conditioning is so pervasive in our society that even someone trying to do real harm will often resort to these sorts of tactics. They generally involve bludgeoning blows from the fists, arms or legs, or grabs, locks and chokes designed to control or suffocate an opponent without causing real harm, or at least not the kind of harm that can be caused just as easily with less effort.

14

Instinctively we know how to fight much more effectively than this, we know how to truly bring our claws out and use our most effective weapons to attack our opponent's most vulnerable targets (more details of how to do this are found in later chapters of this book). This may initially be distasteful to us, possibly causing us to physically and psychologically recoil. In fact because of our social conditioning many people will physically recoil even as they are striking their opponent. This greatly slows down the strike, reducing its power and efficacy, and increases the likelihood of injuring ourselves. This same conditioning may cause us to 'freeze' up at the time we most need to act, as the part of our brain responsible for instinctive action struggles with the conflict between preserving ourselves and continuing to 'be nice' and not harm others.

When we strike it is important for maximum effectiveness that we put our whole mind and body into it without restriction.

It helps if we can logically address in our own minds the concerns we may have about harming another person. Remember the conditioning against this is strong and deep, beginning in our earliest childhood and continuing throughout our lives.

When someone chooses to attack us, they are acting outside the rules of our civilized society. They are acting like an animal. Usually when someone attacks us it will be because they expect to win, probably easily. Much like the dog which attacks a cat, our opponent will likely be bigger, stronger, better armed, more highly skilled, or even acting as part of a group. They are attacking us because they expect to get away with it without incurring much, if any, harm on their part.

Their intentions may be obvious to us, or not. At the outset it is difficult to tell what the outcome of such a situation will be, but once we put ourselves under our attacker's control, once we lose the ability to fight back, we don't really know what the end results will be. They could include serious injury, rape, death, perhaps even death or harm to our loved ones.

While our society's rules have trained us to be nonviolent in most situations, they do not require us to subject ourselves to this.

The time to stop these things from happening is at the outset by acting decisively. Our first preference is always to simply escape the situation along with our loved ones. In many instances though, this will not be a viable option. The attack may be too sudden. We may find ourselves cornered. Or we, or someone under our care, may not physically be able to outrun or escape our attacker. This will often mean we need to harm our attacker physically, possibly seriously, in order to protect ourselves.

The responsibility for this lies on the attacker's shoulders. They chose this path when they violated the rules of our civilized society and reverted to the law of the jungle. If we hold back from defending ourselves because we are afraid of inflicting damage on them, we are allowing them to inflict the same or worse consequences on us or our loved ones. We are also allowing them to potentially carry out further violence on others in future situations. You don't have to do that. You don't want to do that. You don't need to do that.

The health and safety of you, your family and loved ones comes first.

When the time comes, give yourself permission to set loose your INNER TIGER.

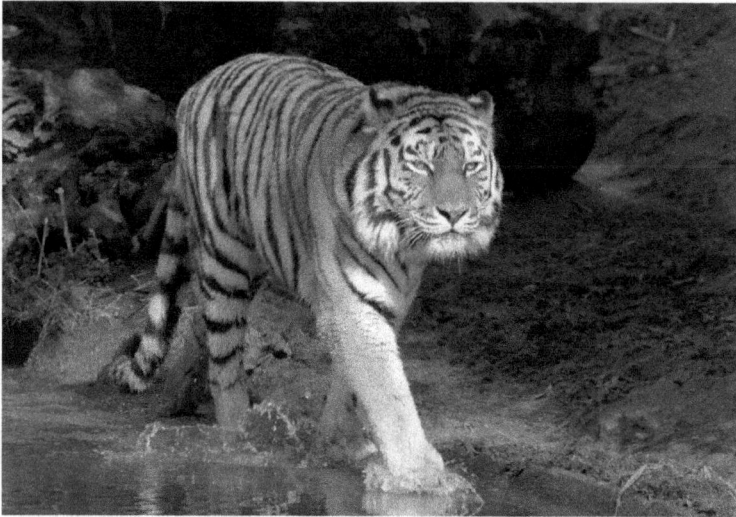

Note on using reasonable force:

It is important to become familiar with the laws around self defense in the legal jurisdiction you live in.

In the jurisdiction I am familiar with, the test is whether you honestly feel under threat. If you do not feel threatened there is no need to use violence. If you do not think a serious threat is posed, but there is still a threat – you may use more moderate force to defend yourself. For myself as a 6 foot 4 inch, 220 pound male with significant martial arts training, the threshold at which I would feel threatened and therefore be justified in using effective violence against an opponent is quite high. If however you are female, significantly smaller than your attacker, are outnumbered, the attacker has a weapon etc; that threshold is a lot lower.

The point where you no longer feel under threat is the point at which you are no longer justified in using violence against your attacker. This may mean that your opponent has backed off, that your opponent is clearly incapacitated, or an opportunity has arisen for you to safely leave the situation.

Chapter Three: Lessons from a cat

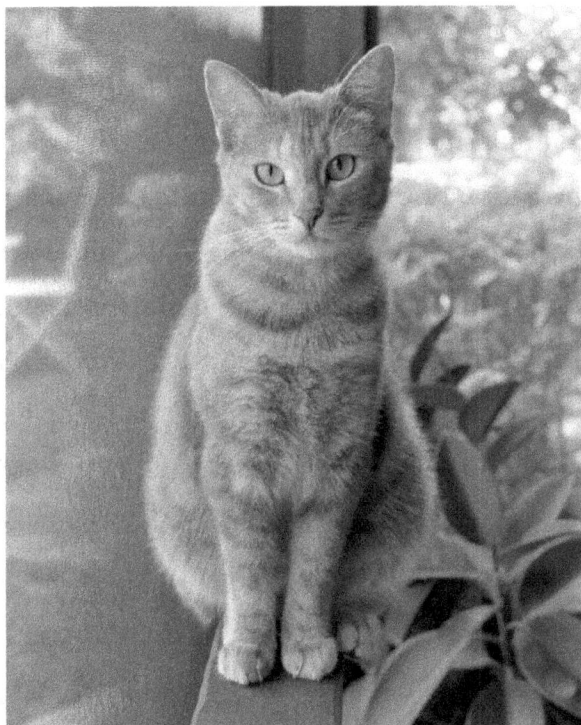

The Chinese martial arts have a long history of observing animals and applying the lessons learned to fighting techniques. Usually the animals observed are in the wild and they are copied both for the economy of motion, the power they produce, the tactics they use in a fight and also their 'spirit' – the drive that helps them to surmount whatever odds they face.

These martial arts usually take years of diligent practice and hard physical and mental training to master, conferring on the practitioner amazing fighting skills and physical abilities much like the animals emulated. For most of us this is not a practical option. In our civilized society it is important for us to put our time, attention and resources into other pursuits. Our lives are more like that of a domestic house cat than a tiger living in the wild, so it makes sense to learn from the example of the domesticated cat that still manages to beat off the attack of a much larger dog. This cat manages to live and act in a way conducive to the civilized environment in which it finds itself yet still retain enough of its wild past, its 'inner tiger' to keep itself safe when it needs to. We can learn not only from what it does in the moment of the attack, but also from the preparations the cat has made long before any kind of attack occurs.

You see, the cat with an inner tiger is confident, not stupid. It doesn't go seeking fights with larger aggressive opponents. Quite the opposite, it does everything it can to avoid such a situation in the first place by being aware of its environment and alert to the situation around it. It prepares for the worst, but acts in such a way that minimizes the likelihood that it will ever need to use the skills it has developed. These preparations leave the cat confident and calm, able to go about its daily activities without worry or fear.

Some of the lessons we can learn from this cat are listed below:

1. The cat with an inner tiger carefully stakes out its territory. It will proceed into a new environment with caution, scanning carefully as it enters, making sure to identify any potential threats, also identifying escape routes if necessary (even a tiger knows that sometimes it is best to beat a retreat).

2. The cat with an inner tiger remains alert to all that goes on around it. You will see it periodically pricking up its ears, keeping an eye half open, maybe even raising its head and having a look around every now and then so it is aware of anyone coming or going.

3. The cat with an inner tiger is a good judge of character and mood. It practices observing those around it so that it can easily identify any new threat at the earliest possible moment. This cat then avoids the threat if possible.

4.   The cat with an inner tiger uses its presence, its voice and body language, to maximum effect to undermine the confidence of its attacker, often avoiding the need for further violence.

5.   The cat with an inner tiger knows which of its weapons are most effective, and knows how to use them, it attacks with its teeth and claws (a tiger will generally not attempt to defeat its foes by lashing its tail at them).

6.   The cat with an inner tiger knows its opponent's weakest most sensitive areas and directs its attacks at these areas getting maximum results with a minimum amount of time and effort.

7.   The cat with an inner tiger practices using its weapons. You'll see it stalking birds, playing with string, scratching bark on trees (or your furniture).

8.   The cat with an inner tiger, on a day to day basis is just a regular, happy, relaxed cat.

Each of these lessons will be examined in subsequent chapters. Read them carefully and do the exercises as you go so that you too can go about your life alert, aware, and confident like a cat.

Chapter Four: Staking out your territory

Have you ever watched a cat as it enters a new territory? It might be crossing your backyard for the first time on its way somewhere else. It might be being introduced to a new house when its owners have moved.

The cat will generally be very cautious at first. It will take it's time, look around, listen very carefully, sniff the air, maybe sniff some of the furniture. It will start at the edges and proceed cautiously out towards the middle of the area, looking around corners.

What is the cat doing?

It is getting the lie of the land. It is checking first for exits or safe havens in case it needs them. It is amazing how quickly a cat can turn and dash up the nearest tree or over the nearest fence when it needs to.

It is checking for any threats that may be in the area, it is also smelling and listening carefully in case there has been a potential threat there in the past, or there may be one nearby that may return soon.

Once the cat has made its initial assessment of both the immediate area and its surroundings, it will relax and start to look for other things of interest to it – food, playthings. It may even curl up and take a nap. Now it knows its options, it knows it is safe for the time being and has formulated a plan of where it can go if a threat does enter this new territory. It is more relaxed than if it had not taken the time to survey its surroundings because now it knows it is unlikely to have a nasty surprise. If it does, it has contingency plans in place which it can act on in an instant.

You will notice that when the cat then comes back to the same environment, even one it has lived in for years, it will pause, just briefly and look around before proceeding about its business. It already knows its options, it is just checking in case anything has changed, or a new threat has emerged.

Think about some of the environments you are in on a regular basis. If there were a threat, where would it most likely come from? Where could you go if you needed to get away? Where could you go to get help in a hurry or let someone know you are in trouble? Is there any way that you could get advanced warning of an approaching threat?

These are some simple steps you can take to know your options and help you relax in any given environment. This is very important. You are learning self defense, not so that you can live a life of worry and fear, but so that you can live a life of confidence and enjoyment.

Exercise 2:

Take some time now to think about your home, your workplace, your transportation, and any other places you go regularly.

Answer the following questions:

1. **What possible threats are there in this environment?** *At home, possible threats could be an intruder, someone who is already in the house when you arrive home, or someone who breaks in while you are already there. It could also be a friend or acquaintance. At work a threat could come from customers or co-workers. On the street a threat could come from almost anyone.*

   If you feel the environment is too dangerous, you can ask yourself: Do I really need to be here? Sometimes the best option is to simply not go somewhere that

*contains too significant a threat, or leave that place
as soon as you can.*

2.   ***Where would these threats most likely come from?***
      *Would a threat come through your door? Your
      window? From the other side of the counter? From
      around a corner? From behind you?*

3.   ***What exits are available?*** *What are ALL the
      available exits? Doors, windows, gates, paths,
      climbable fences and walls? If a threat comes from
      one direction, what options are left available?
      Which is the best and easiest exit?*

4.   ***Where can you go as a safe haven nearby? Or is
      there anyone nearby that could come to your aid,
      and how would you let them know you need it?*** *Is
      there someone else in the house that you can go to or
      yell for? Do you have neighbors you can trust and
      reach easily? Can you get to a co-worker's office?
      On the street, are there any security guards nearby?
      Is there a convenience store or other business nearby
      where you can go for help? If you scream will
      someone hear you? What should you yell to get the
      quickest response?*

Do this for each of the environments you find yourself in regularly; then practice making a similar analysis whenever you go somewhere new.

Several examples are included below.

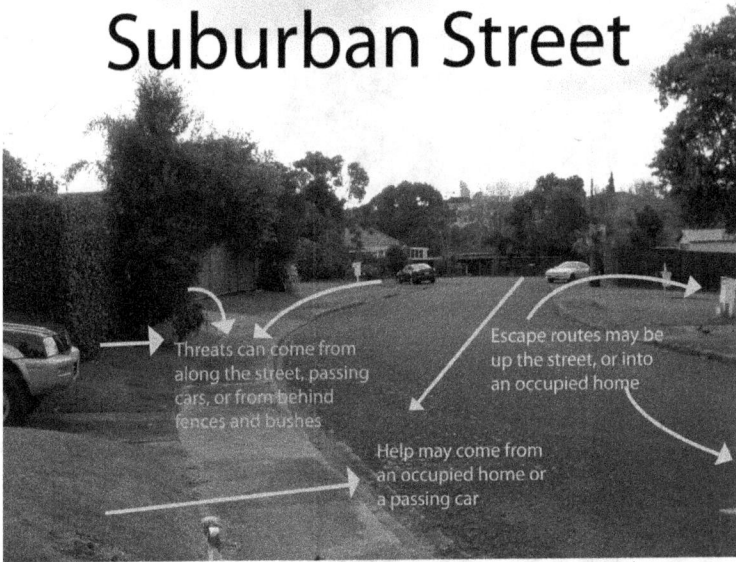

Suburban Street

Threats can come from along the street, passing cars, or from behind fences and bushes

Escape routes may be up the street, or into an occupied home

Help may come from an occupied home or a passing car

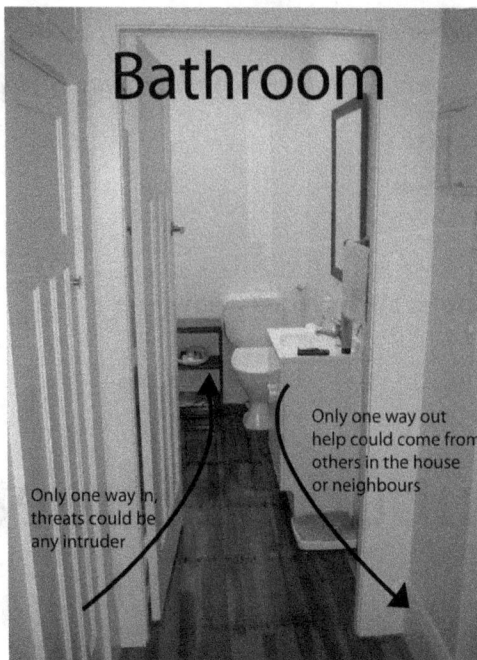

Bathroom

Only one way out
help could come from
others in the house
or neighbours

Only one way in,
threats could be
any intruder

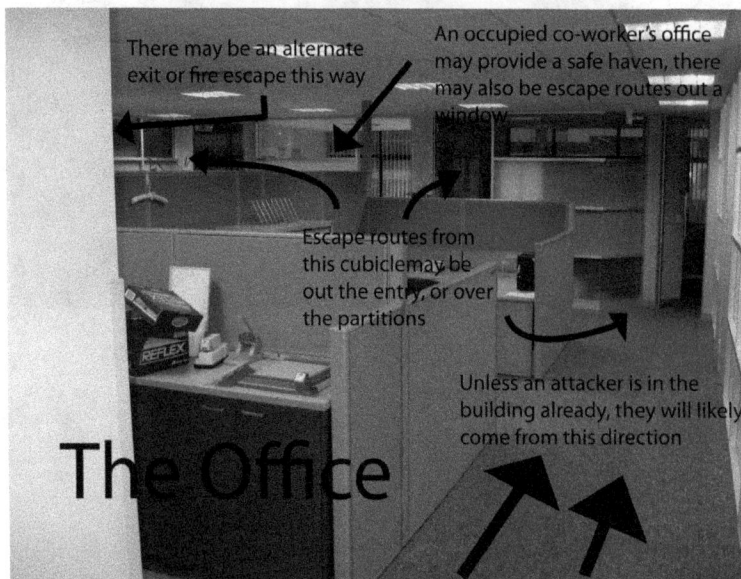

There may be an alternate
exit or fire escape this way

An occupied co-worker's office
may provide a safe haven, there
may also be escape routes out a
window

Escape routes from
this cubicle may be
out the entry, or over
the partitions

Unless an attacker is in the
building already, they will likely
come from this direction

The Office

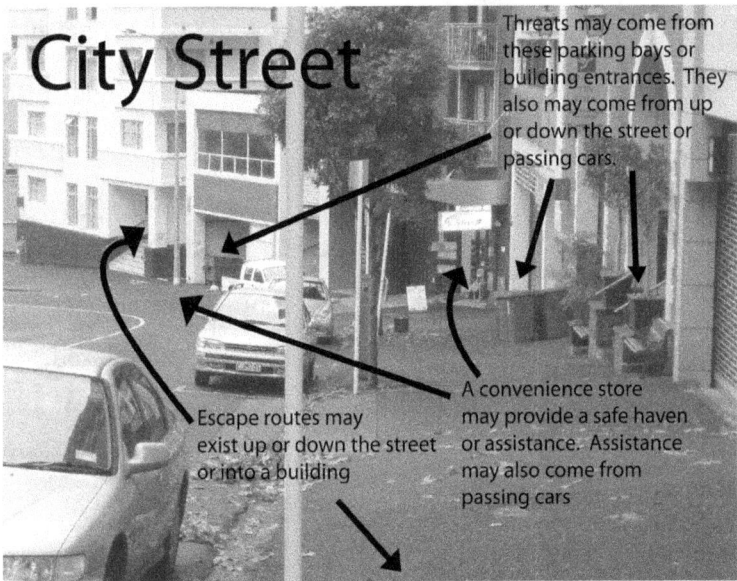

City Street

Threats may come from these parking bays or building entrances. They also may come from up or down the street or passing cars.

A convenience store may provide a safe haven or assistance. Assistance may also come from passing cars

Escape routes may exist up or down the street or into a building

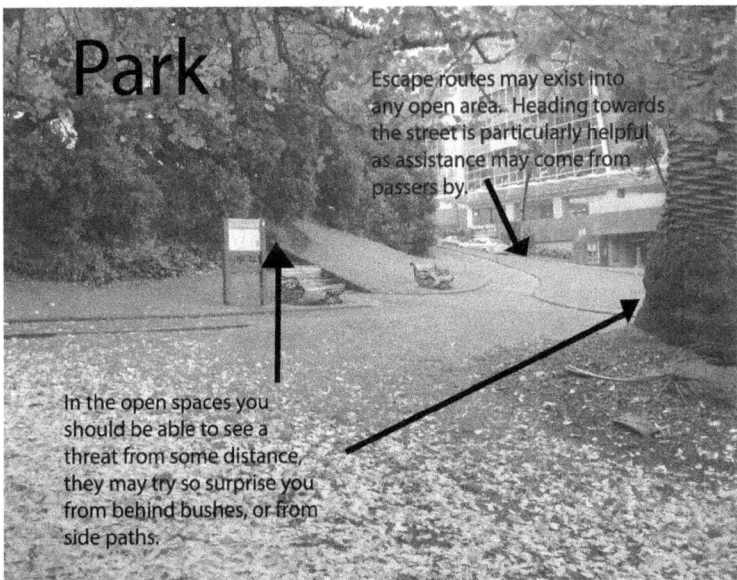

Park

Escape routes may exist into any open area. Heading towards the street is particularly helpful as assistance may come from passers by.

In the open spaces you should be able to see a threat from some distance, they may try so surprise you from behind bushes, or from side paths.

If you do this regularly you will soon get into the habit and become faster and faster at making your analysis. You can even make it a game with your friends while you are getting used to it. Before long you will do it automatically, quickly and unconsciously.

Remember the object of this exercise is not to make you nervous, tense or paranoid. Quite the opposite. Being prepared will help you to be calm, confident and relaxed, leaving you free to enjoy yourself and get on with the things you want to do.

Chapter Five: Remaining alert

After a cat has staked out its territory, new or familiar, it
will get on with its usual business, maybe even taking a nap.
But you will notice even as the cat lies snoozing in the sun,
every now and then its ears will twitch and maybe stand up
for awhile. The cat may half open an eye every once in
awhile, and if it sees, hears or even smells something it is
not sure about, it will lift it's head and ears right up,
craning it's neck for a better look or listen until it is
satisfied that the situation is still safe.

The cat is using all of its senses so that it can become aware
of any threats at the earliest possible moment, giving it
more time to respond should the need arise.

In practical terms for us this means remaining alert to what
is going on around us, and putting strategies in place to
give us advance warning of a possible threat.

For example, in your home, do you have a security system,
alarms or cameras? Do you use them? Do you lock your
doors and windows? A lock will not keep a determined

intruder out, but it will give you advanced notice of their entry.

Do you take a moment every now and then to look up from your work or whatever you are doing and observe what is going on around you?

In your office, do you sit with your back to the door? Can you sit so you can see anyone entering? If not, can you place a mirror or even some other shiny reflective object on your desk, that will let you know, either consciously or unconsciously, of any movement behind you?

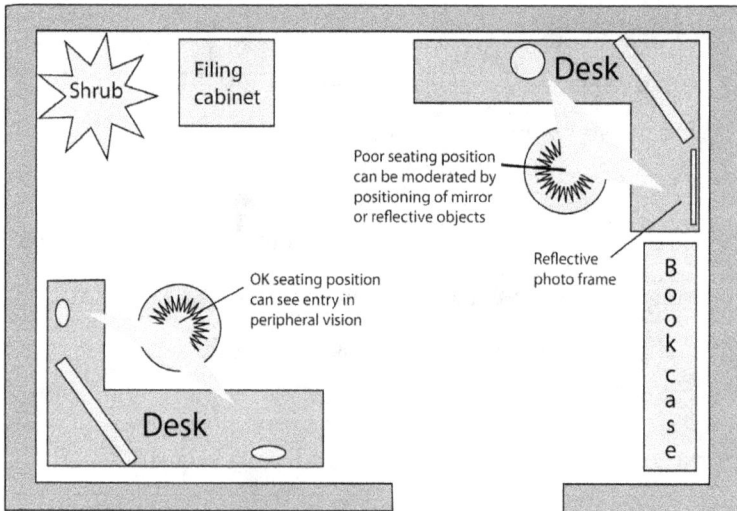

When you are out, can you position yourself in a way that makes it difficult for someone to sneak up behind you? Perhaps placing something solid such as a wall behind you, or if you are with a group, positioning yourself so that if you can't see behind yourself, someone else in your group can.

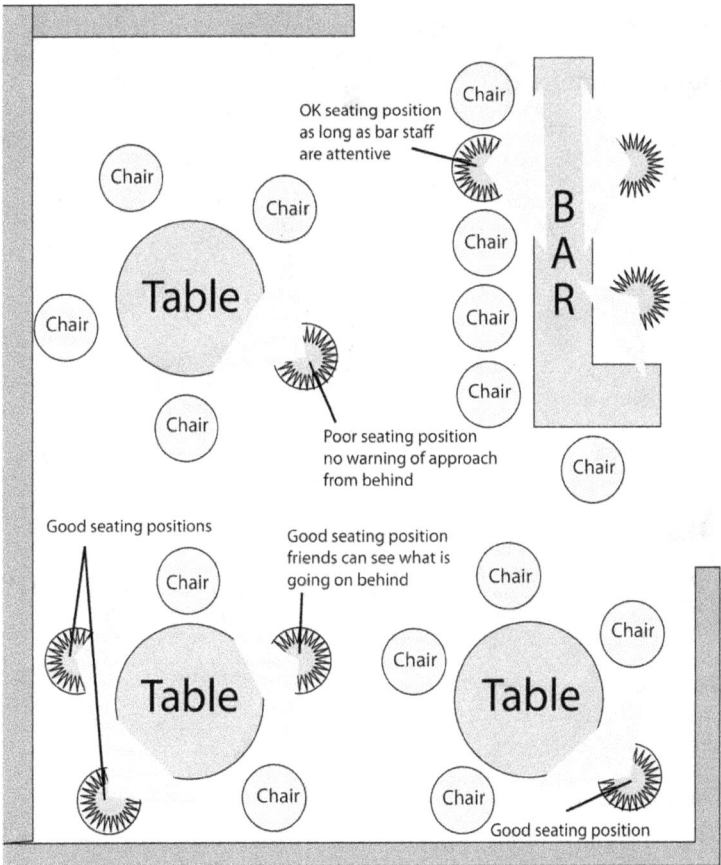

OK seating position as long as bar staff are attentive

Poor seating position no warning of approach from behind

Good seating positions

Good seating position friends can see what is going on behind

Good seating position

Exercise 3:

Take a few moments to consider the environments you are frequently in. What steps can you take to allow yourself advanced warning of the approach of a possible threat?

Practice taking simple steps such as these, and it will quickly become a habit. You will be more aware of what is going on around you, and more confident and in control of your environment.

Chapter Six: Identifying a threat

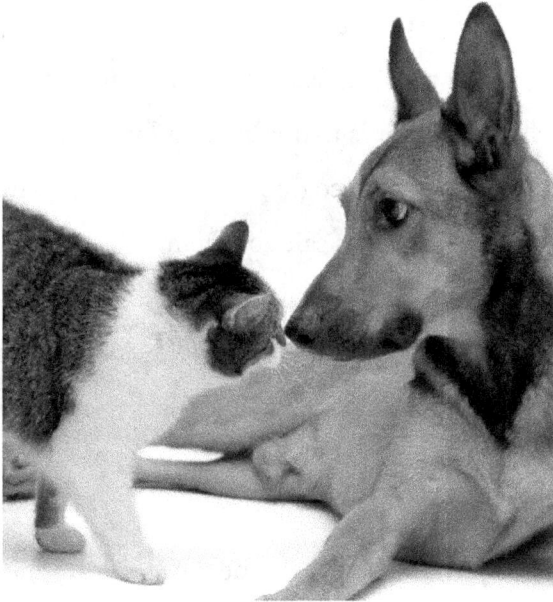

Have you ever watched a cat walk right up to someone it doesn't know and rub itself against their legs, yet stay away from someone else? Or have you seen a cat go right up to a large dog and rub against it or touch noses?

How does the cat know who will receive it well and who to stay clear of? How does it know a friendly dog from a mean one?

The cat has probably observed the person or animal from a distance, using all of its senses to get a gauge of what they are like, what kind of mood they are in, and what their attitudes and actions are likely to be. The cat listens to their footsteps and voice, smells their sweat, and of course visually observes physical features and posture. A cat will generally know who it is that is coming long before they actually arrive. If they recognize them, they will have a good idea of whether it is safe for them to be around them or not. If the cat does not recognize them it will either approach cautiously or make a judgment call based on past experience with other people or animals displaying similar attributes.

Whenever my young nieces and nephews are around, my cat is mysteriously nowhere to be seen. Not because the children are going to intentionally hurt him, but because he doesn't particularly enjoy 'hugs' and other rather rough signs of affection that small children like to give to animals. He also tends to make himself scarce whenever other small children are around, as he has learned that they are likely to display the same type of behavior. When they are gone he suddenly re-appears.

The people the cat approaches safely are not always the ones that are well groomed or good looking. It's not always the biggest toughest looking dogs the cat stays away from.

The cat has become an expert in human and animal behavior. It has learned to use all its senses to read moods and attitudes and make an accurate assessment of risk long before actually coming into contact with another animal or human.

We can learn these same skills.

<u>Exercise 4:</u>

Take time out once in awhile to do some people watching. Do it discretely, in many cultures it is impolite to stare. Try it in different locations, as you are eating lunch in a cafeteria, waiting at the traffic lights in your car, in a business meeting. Look at people's posture. Look at the way they respond to things. Listen to the tone of their voice. When observing from a distance, try to tell what is going on between people even when you can't hear what they are saying.

Do this for awhile and you will begin to notice patterns, the slight changes in posture and gesture that show that a girl is really interested in a guy, or just being polite. The tone of voice that lets you know that someone is holding something back. Even that little something you can't quite put your finger on, that lets you know something isn't right in a situation.

Many of us do this unconsciously already. Take some time to practice consciously though and your skills will improve greatly.

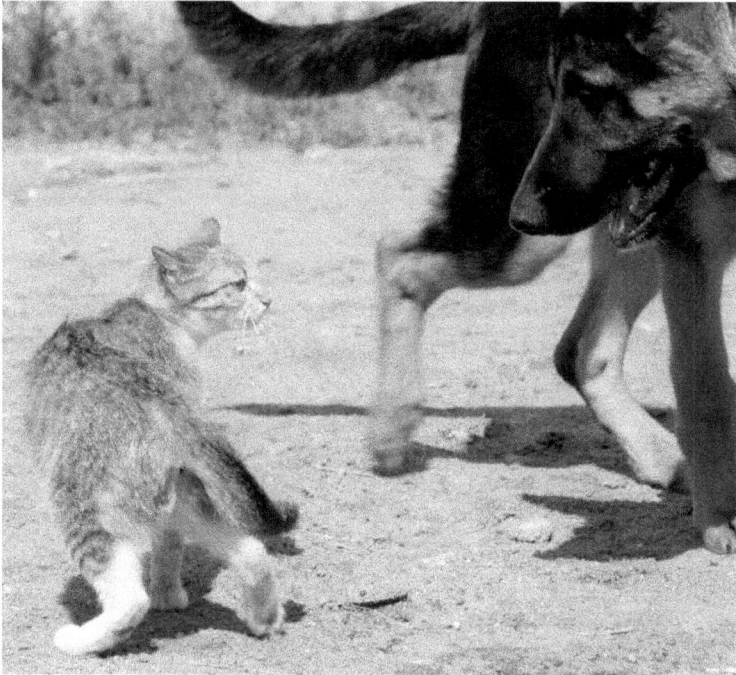

There are some specific warning signs it can be helpful to look out for:

The smell of alcohol or drugs on the breath or clothes. People in an intoxicated state often do things that they would not normally do.

Excessively dilated or constricted pupils. Shifty eyes that will not focus or continue to look in unexpected directions. The eyes are the window to the soul... they also tell you a lot about how the central nervous system is functioning. Excessive dilation or constriction can be a sign of an extreme emotional state or of mind-altering drug consumption. The attention generally follows the gaze, and someone who keeps shifting their focus may be trying to hide their intentions.

People who pretend they haven't noticed you when it is obvious they have. Again they may be attempting to conceal their intentions.

People who approach closer to you than social norms would dictate in a particular situation, particularly when there is no-one else around.

As you practice you will begin to notice more and more about the people around you. Do not make assumptions based on your assessments, but use them to help guide your actions. Someone you have a bad feeling about may not in fact be a predator, but may be having a bad day, perhaps dealing with personal problems or even have a medical condition. Do not judge them because of this, but do take sensible precautions.

When in doubt about someone, politely stay away or approach with caution. If you have to spend time around someone you do not feel comfortable with, is there some way you can keep a safe distance between you and them? Can you go somewhere there are other people around that you trust? Can you simply observe them a little more closely than normal until you come to grips with what to expect from them?

The best way to avoid a threat is to try to never put yourself in a situation where you are alone with someone who might pose one to you.

Chapter Seven: Establishing your presence

Have you ever been near a real live tiger? Even when the tiger is calm it has a presence that dominates a room. When it becomes angry, or wants to warn others away, the effect becomes undeniable. Every part of its body is involved as it exudes power and authority. The tiger cannot be ignored and commands the respect of all around it.

A domestic cat which brings out its inner tiger uses the same principles when under threat to let its attacker know just what it is dealing with. The cat will turn and face the attacking dog head on. It will arch its back and bristle its fur. Its face will change from calm and placid to fierce and angry. It will hiss. Every part of its body is engaged, both preparing for action and letting the attacker know it may be getting more than it bargained for. Often just these actions alone are enough to make the dog reconsider and back off.

We can use similar principles when we find ourselves under threat.

This begins with how we go about our daily activities. If we go about feeling calm, confident, and aware, this will carry over into our posture and body language. Subtle changes in the way you carry yourself, the way you hold your head, the expression on your face, even your tone of voice, let others around you know that you are comfortable and able to take care of yourself. Going through the exercises in this book and mentally and physically preparing yourself will give you this natural inner confidence.

This makes it less likely that a predator will approach you randomly as they will generally go after the easiest target they can find. You are not an easy target!

Of course you may still find yourself targeted simply by being in the wrong place at the wrong time, or when a predator has other strong motives.

When this occurs, the first step is to turn and face the potential threat, both physically and psychologically. Hopefully you will be able to anticipate the potential threat before they actually reach you. If this happens as well as turning and looking directly at the threat, you can loudly and firmly address the potential threat, questioning what they are doing and telling them not to do it if you feel uncomfortable.

This does three things:

It lets the potential threat know you are aware of them and what they are doing.

It lets the potential threat know that you are no push over. You are willing to stick up for yourself and oppose what you are uncomfortable with.

If others are around, it draws their attention to what is going on.

This is very off putting to a predator as they now face:

Having lost any element of surprise they thought they had.

The knowledge that they can expect resistance.

An increased possibility of intervention by others.

And of course, it may be possible that you have misread someone's intentions. They may not have you in mind as a target, and this gives an innocent party the opportunity to modify their actions or leave the area. It also gives a true predator the opportunity to back off without further repercussions as they have not yet incriminated themselves, so they are not committed to following through on any intentions they may have had.

If after this the threat persists, your physical transformation begins. This is the time you want your body to switch on. You WANT your 'fight or flight' response to kick in. You WANT your body to release adrenalin, your pupils to dilate, blood and energy to rush to your muscles. Remember you can choose how this 'fight or flight' response manifests, whether it be as fear, anger or just alert determination.

Exercise 5:

Set your legs at least shoulder width apart, one foot slightly in front of the other. Lower your centre of gravity by bending your knees slightly. Relax your shoulders. Bring your hands and arms up in front of your body facing towards your opponent. This is a confident posture, ready for action.

Widen you eyes, clench you jaw, let your face take on a fierce look. We've all heard of the 'eye of the tiger', now is the time to use it. All these changes will occur naturally and quickly and are as much or more about what we are thinking internally as what is going on with the position of our body parts. The body is simply reflecting what is going on in the mind.

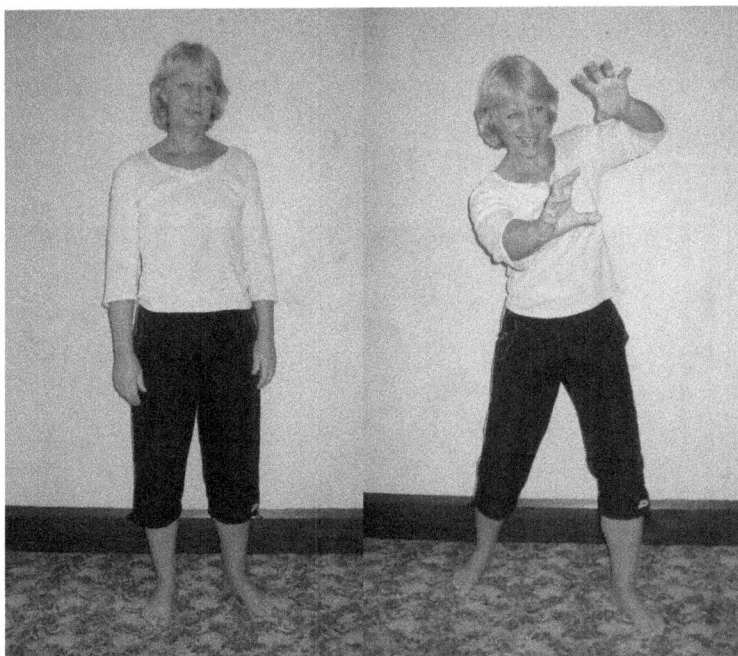

Of course it helps if your body has had at least some practice assuming this kind of look, as it will feel more familiar and natural. You can practice this in front of mirror if you want. It may feel awkward at first, or you may feel a little funny. In fact it is good to have fun with it. Enjoy seeing just how fierce you can make yourself look. It helps if you have something you can say to yourself inside to reinforce this fierce attitude. It could be something like "you're mine!" "bring it on!" or "get ready for pain". Experiment and find something that suits you. You can

even take it further and imagine you ARE a TIGER! Imagine
your body is loose, fast and strong like a tiger's. Imagine your
hands are powerful claws. Imagine your teeth are fangs. Your
fur bristles when an opponent approaches and your face takes on
the fierce face of an angry cat with eyes glaring as you anticipate
action!

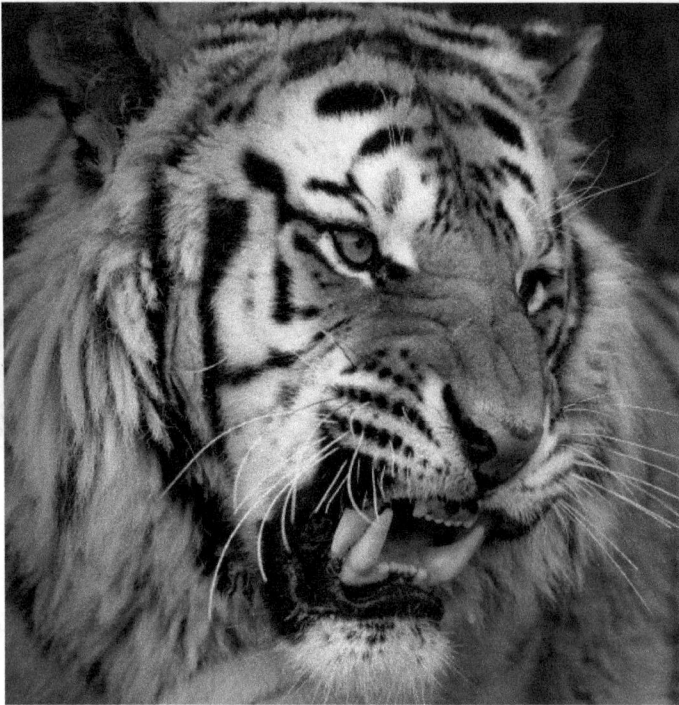

Imagine your opponents surprise when the gentle, helpless
looking little domestic cat he or she was going to attack
transforms into a FIERCE TIGER right in front of his or
her eyes!!!

This is often enough to cause a predator to rethink his or her actions, or at least take the confidence out of their movements as they lose their fighting spirit.

Chapter Eight: The claws come out

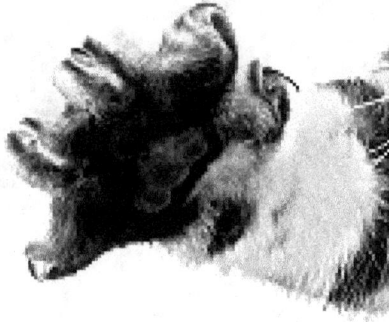

When a tiger attacks it uses its best weapons; its claws, its teeth. Only when it's playing does it use its paws without using the claws as well.

As humans we have a huge arsenal of effective weapons we can use against an opponent, some of which are more effective than others. When we think of an arsenal of weapons we often think of something like this:

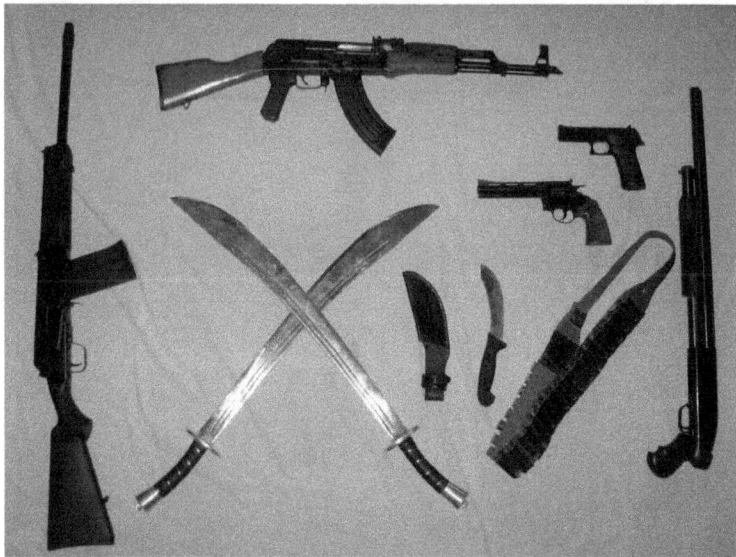

These are good weapons, but most of us are unlikely to have access to these types of weapons when we are faced with an attack.

We will often have access to a range of other weapons. This is an arsenal of weapons we may be carrying on us right now:

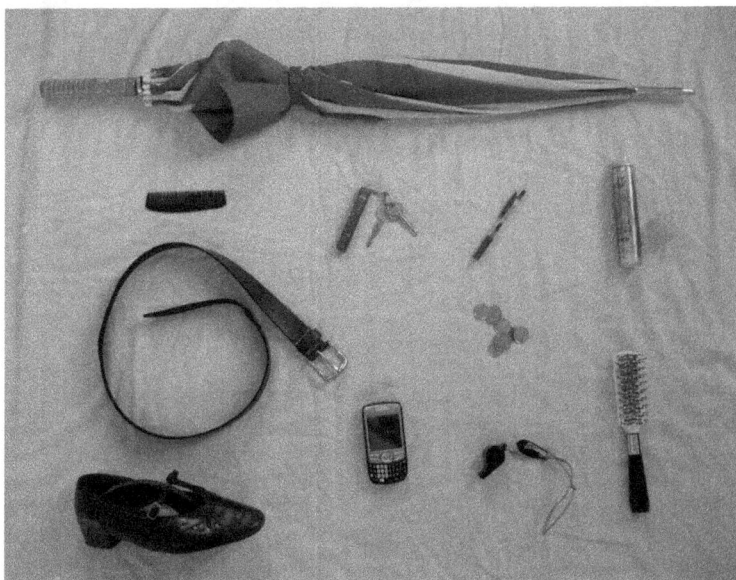

We call these weapons of opportunity. Items that serve other purposes that can be picked up and used effectively as a weapon at a moments notice. An effective weapon is anything that is hard or has pointy bits that we can grasp and swing easily. It is anything that extends our reach. It is also anything that is heavy and solid or anything that causes enough irritation to seriously impair the senses.

Hairspray or deodorant can be sprayed in the eyes to blind and distract your opponent. A whistle can be blown loudly, both to attract attention and if done close enough to the ear of an opponent, to cause pain and disorientation. The hard points of car keys, the handle of a comb, the end of a pen, the corner of a cellphone can be thrust into or slashed across sensitive areas. A heeled shoe can be stomped into an opponents foot or other exposed areas. An umbrella can be thrust into an opponent, keeping them at bay.

There may be other weapons which you can grab easily nearby:

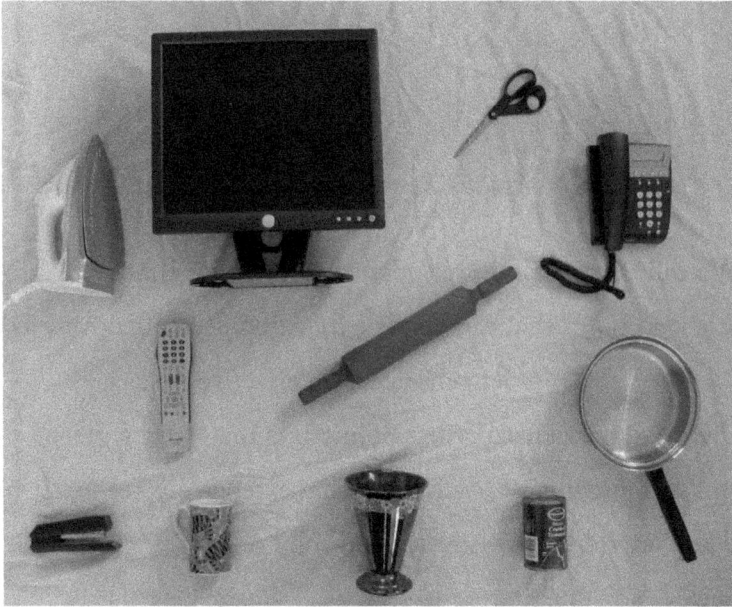

Anything hard, such as a telephone can be swung with good effect against the body. When it has more weight such as a vase, frying pan or computer screen we need to make sure our first strike with it is a good one, we may only get one strike as we will move more slowly with a heavy object than with a light one. We can throw hot drinks in the face of an attacker, obscuring their vision.

Of course there are many other items around us every day which can make good weapons. Be creative and practice identifying potential weapons in any environment you find yourself in.

Exercise 6:

Take a moment to go through the items you have on your person at the moment. Which of them would make a good weapon? How easily and quickly can you get hold of and use these weapons?

Now look around the environment you are in now. What items can you see that would make good weapons? How easily could you reach and use them if you needed to?

Practice this exercise from time to time in any of the environments you frequently find yourself in.

There may of course be times when we do not have access even to these, in which case we use the arsenal of weapons we carry with us as parts of our bodies.

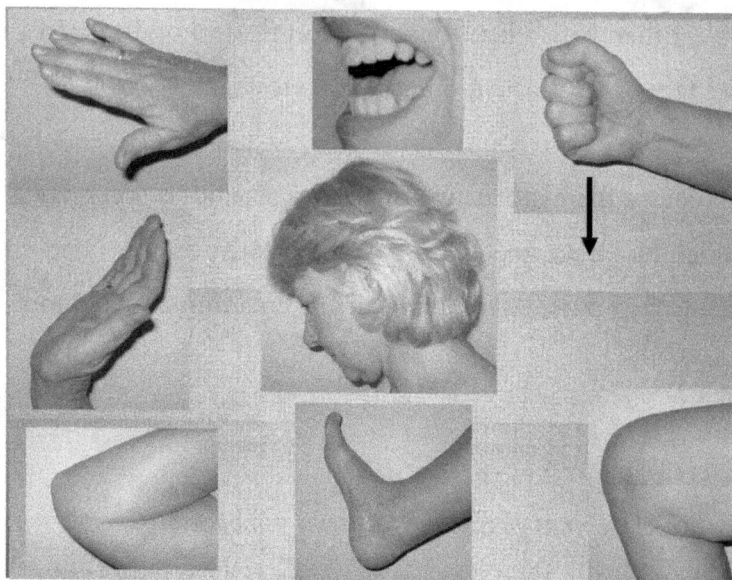

You will notice that next to the picture of a fist there is an arrow pointing downwards. This indicates that this weapon is to be swung downwards like a hammer. Unless you have learned to strike with individual knuckles a regular fist is essentially a bludgeoning weapon. To throw it straight out with significant force takes training and practice, and even then trained professional fighters will often break knuckles or wrists using these types of blows and they have spent years working with these strikes. The regular fist has developed through sporting application when we both literally and metaphorically put the 'gloves on'. When we use these fists, generally we are not trying to seriously damage our opponent, simply beat him or her in a contest and show our dominance. Our bodies have other weapons which we can use more effectively with less chance of injury to ourselves.

The heel of the hand can take the place of the regular fist for many of these linear striking movements. It is very hard and unlikely to be injured when we are striking our opponent. It also allows the fingertips to rapidly be brought to bear on any sensitive areas which are exposed.

A hammer fist is useful as we can still use it as a bludgeoning weapon except this time we swing it much like a hammer, a movement which is easy to learn and instinctive to use. The hammer fist makes the hand tight and compact and we are far less likely to injure our hands striking with the side of our fists in this way.

The tips of our fingers are an excellent weapon, thrusting, gripping into and slashing across sensitive areas, especially if we have tough fingernails.

Our bent knees and elbows and the heels of our feet are very hard and can be brought to bear with great force. The elbows and heels are particularly good when our opponent is behind us. We can elbow backwards into the ribs or head and stomp down into the feet and shins.

We can even use our head as a weapon. Bring it down onto something soft and sensitive like the nose, or bite at whatever we can reach. Screaming and yelling with our mouths will draw attention and possibly aid, and can also act as a weapon if we do it close enough to our attacker's ear.

By the using the best weapons we have available against our opponent's most vulnerable targets, even the smallest of us can beat off a very large attacker. Use your best weapons first.

Chapter Nine: The hunter becomes the hunted

Violent confrontations are unpredictable. The longer they go on, the more likely it is that someone will become seriously hurt, injured or even killed. It can be as simple as someone being knocked down and hitting their head on something hard on the way down. I personally know a man who killed his uncle with one punch during a heated argument. He had no intention of killing his uncle, but it happened anyway as a result of the situation turning violent.

Violence should never be taken lightly. When someone attacks you, they are putting you at risk of these sorts of consequences. You also do not know what intentions they may have for you once they have you under their control.

When we are placed in a situation where we are under significant physical threat and have to use violence to protect ourselves or others, our aim is to get out of the situation as quickly as possible. We do this by attacking our opponent in as ferocious and effective a manner as we possibly can until our opponent is no longer a threat either due to having left the area, backed off to such an extent that we are able to leave safely, or having become incapacitated. This can also allow us to deal with multiple attackers by quickly dispatching each of them individually.

The key is to remember we have now returned to the law of the jungle. Our attacker has put us back there by acting like an animal and instigating violence against us. We are the TIGER in this situation and our opponent is our prey. The hunter has become the hunted. Our aim is to deal with the threat as quickly and effectively as possible to minimize the chance of harm to ourselves.

We do this by striking immediately and repeatedly for our opponent's most sensitive areas in rapid succession, using the best weapons we have available to us at the time. We put our whole body, energy and emotion into this. We overwhelm our opponent with the suddenness and ferocity of the attack, inflicting as much damage and pain as we can immediately, not stopping until we are no longer at risk. By doing this we psychologically turn the tables on our opponent. Our opponent thought they were the hunter. They were going to inflict violence on us their prey. Suddenly they are confronted with a very different reality. One in which they are experiencing pain and a rapid, bewildering onslaught of attack. It is their turn to take fright.

They probably have not prepared themselves for this, and if they have not programmed effective responses to this into their brain and nervous system, it is likely that their reactions will slow, at least momentarily as they adapt to the new situation. When we attack in this way we increase our chances of landing a strike somewhere with enough force to physically incapacitate our opponent, bringing the conflict to an end. We also increase the likelihood that our attacker will back off, either turning tail and running, or at least retreating enough to give us a good opportunity to escape safely, much like the dog attacking the domestic cat in our story.

In order to do this effectively we need to think objectively about our opponent's body. We need to know the areas that are most sensitive and vulnerable to damage. The areas that when hit, will cause the most pain, impairment and distraction possible. These are the areas we will strike at.

Below is a map of the human body with a list of sensitive targets and how to attack them. The sensitive areas for males and females are identical apart from testicles in men and breasts in women, these areas are covered in the notes which follow:

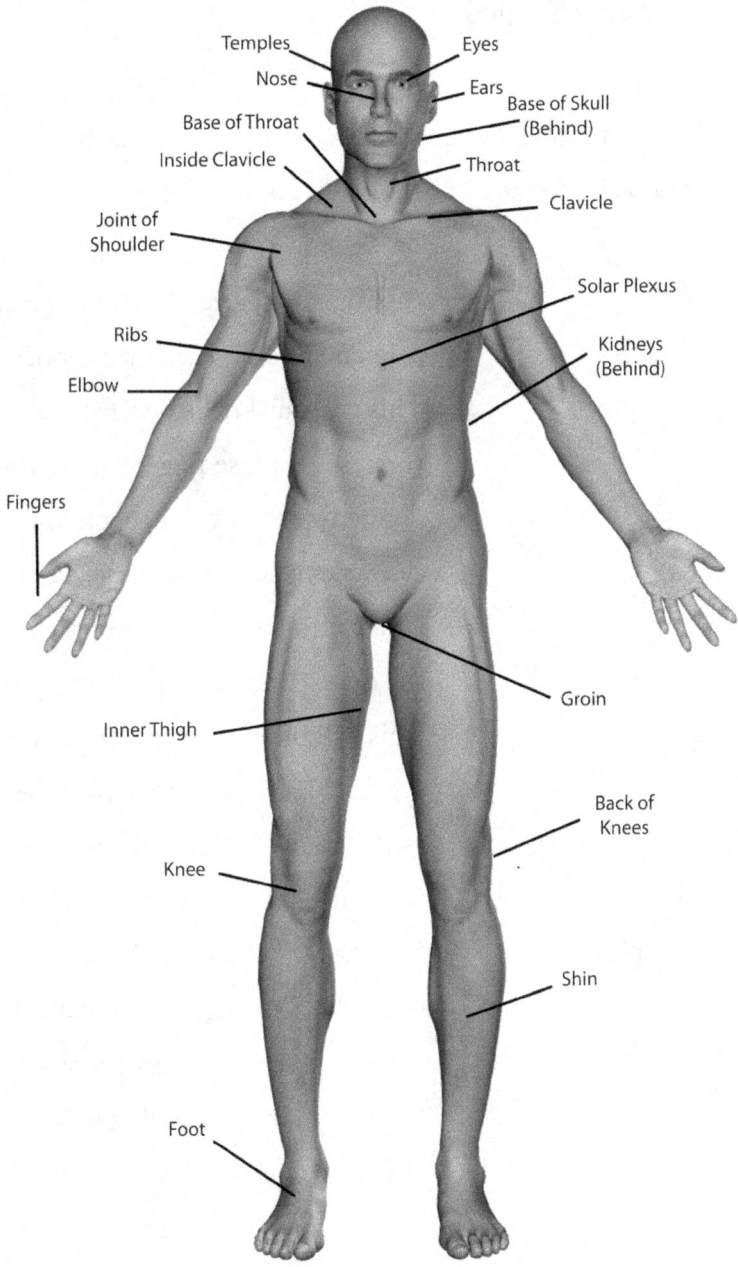

Temples

Eyes

Nose

Ears

Base of Skull
(Behind)

Base of Throat

Inside Clavicle

Throat

Joint of
Shoulder

Clavicle

Solar Plexus

Ribs

Kidneys
(Behind)

Elbow

Fingers

Groin

Inner Thigh

Back of
Knees

Knee

Shin

Foot

63

Sensitive Targets:

Strikes to the following areas can be lethal or easily cause serious injury, use only if the threat warrants it.

Eyes:

A strike to the eyes will cause great pain and also obscure the vision. This will quickly help to facilitate your escape. Use finger tips or any pointed weapon you happen to have available to slash across the eyes or gouge into them. The eyes are often the easiest and most effective target

Nose:

This will often cause watering in the eyes and blurring of the vision, as well as pain. Strike with any hard weapon.

Temples:

Just above the joint of the jaw. This is the thinnest part of the skull and contains a sensitive nerve centre. Striking with a pointed object such as keys, cellphone or a knuckle will have the greatest effect

Base of Skull:

A hard strike here can cause concussion as the brain stem is

	exposed to the force of the strike. Use any hard weapon.
Ear:	A cupping blow with the palm of your hand across the ear can easily rupture an ear drum, causing great pain and also a loss of balance.
Throat:	A hard blow can crush the windpipe making breathing difficult, or at the very least cause serious pain. Use any hard weapon.

The following areas inflict pain, acting as a distraction and deterrent, serious injury is possible but less likely.

Base of throat:	Striking the hollow at the base of the throat can cause pain and make it difficult to breathe. Use fingers or any pointed weapon.
Inside the Clavicle:	This will cause pain. Use fingers or any pointed weapon.
Joint of the Shoulder:	This will cause pain and can also disable the shoulder joint as it causes damage to the rotator cuff. Use any hard pointed weapon.

Breasts:	Sensitive area on females. Use any weapon. Grab, elbow, kick, knee.
Solar Plexus:	This will cause pain and possibly difficulty breathing. Use any hard weapon. Elbows and knees are particularly good.
Kidneys:	This will cause pain. Use any hard weapon.
Groin:	Particularly the testicles, but also a sensitive area for females. Strikes to this area will cause pain. Use any weapon. Grab, elbow, kick, knee.
Back of the knees:	This will cause pain and also possibly difficulty in pursuing. A great way to take someone down. Kick, stomp or use any hard weapon.
Inner Thigh:	This will cause pain. Susceptible to kicks, also grabs and twists. Particularly useful if someone is on top of you and the testicles are not exposed.
Shin:	This will cause pain, attack with a weapon or stomp downwards with a scraping motion

The following areas can cause pain when struck and also are susceptible to fracture or dislocation, disabling your opponent

Clavicle:	Can break on downward blow. Use any hard heavy weapon.
Elbow:	14 pounds of pressure against a locked elbow will break it. Use any hard heavy weapon
Fingers:	Susceptible to sprains and breaks. Grab and twist hard, bending backwards. Stomp on or bite.
Ribs:	This will cause pain and possibly fractures. Strike here with a solid object or a knee or elbow.
Knee:	Strikes to the inside, outside or front of the knee can be effective. Use any hard, heavy weapon, particularly stomps with the foot.
Foot:	Stomps to the top of the foot will cause pain and may break several small bones in the foot.

Note on dealing with attackers on drugs:

Attackers on certain mind altering substances will not
exhibit the normal responses to pain. They will continue to
attack almost oblivious to any pain inflicted. They may also
exhibit extreme strength, so physical restraint is unlikely to
work unless they can be outnumbered. To effectively deal
with such an attacker, inflicting pain is not enough, they
must be physically incapacitated. This means fracturing
bones or dislocating joints such as the elbow, knee and
shoulder, removing senses such as sight (strikes to the
eyes)and balance (bursting the ear drum), or seriously
reducing oxygen flow to the brain (strikes to the throat).
This is a sad reality in our society today, one that we need
to be prepared to deal with. Remember, reasonable force is
the force necessary for you to escape harm.

Exercise 7:
*Review the chart of sensitive targets. Identify the targets on
your own body touching each area as you go. Practice
identifying the targets on people around you (you don't have to
touch them). Think about how you can effectively strike each
target.*

Chapter Ten: Playing with string

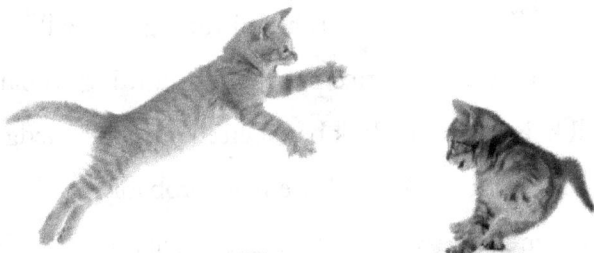

All animals which are natural predators have instinctive behaviors which help them to develop their fighting skills. Young animals will practice stalking each other, insects, and any other small creatures they can find. They will play fight and wrestle together, and once they are older they will hone their skills further by actually hunting.

As humans we have similar natural behaviors, but in our modern society many of us were not permitted to perform them and so our development in this area has been held back. Little kids naturally wrestle and fight with each other, but we were probably told not to because it wasn't "nice", or was "too rough". Many of us probably experienced our parents reacting with horror if we picked up some kind of weapon to play with, toy or otherwise.

This creates great apprehension and even fear of using our natural abilities. As mentioned earlier in this book, this conditioning is strong and deep and it is important that we deal with it in order to react quickly and effectively when we need to. To overcome this conditioning you will probably need some practice playing out fighting scenarios. This will help make the link between mental knowledge and physical action. After all we have probably all viewed acts of violence in movies or on our TV sets, but this doesn't automatically make us into great fighters.

The nervous systems throughout our bodies learn, and having performed movements before will make it easier to perform them again. We will perform them more quickly, confidently and naturally. Of course the more we practice a movement the more efficient and effective we become at it. Exercise physiologists estimate that it takes about 1000 repetitions of a movement for our bodies to truly 'learn' a movement and up to 3000 repetitions to relearn or alter a movement once it has already been learnt. After this the speed, efficiency and power we can generate with that specific movement goes up dramatically. This is great if you have the time and inclination for extensive training. With time and dedication you can develop some truly remarkable skills. Most of us though, have many other demands on our time and priorities of what we want to put our energy into.

The good news is we don't all need to become seasoned fighters and martial artists training in gyms for years on end in order to be able to defend ourselves. What we do need is at least some experience with how it physically feels to be in the type of violent situations we may find ourselves in, and with how we can move and use our bodies in these situations. We may not be a great fighter, or even in great shape, but we can make the most of our current physical abilities by knowing how we can easily strike at our opponent's most sensitive areas with the best weapons we have available. We need practice in figuring out just where we can reach on an opponent's body most easily for greatest effect. Of course the more we practice, the more proficient we will become, but even a short amount of time spent working on this will greatly increase our effectiveness.

A number of specific scenarios and examples of simple effective ways to deal with them follow. You will need to practice these and any other likely scenarios you can think of with a partner.

Be nice to your partner!!

You do not need to actually hit your partner with full force, or scratch them in the eyes, or knee them in the testicles. Always think of the safety of your training partner first.

The examples which follow are by no means the only way to deal with these situations. They are intended to illustrate use of the basic principles. You can and should experiment and come up with many more. The purpose of playing through these situations is not for you to learn set ways of responding but for you to figure out what works best for YOU. When you practice being in any of these types of situation, see where and how you instinctively go to hit immediately. Is it effective? If not try some other options until you come up with something that works. Once you grasp the general principles you will be able to respond creatively and effectively to new situations that may arise.

Run through the movements, slowly at first, more quickly as you gain in confidence. Remember you will be much stronger and faster when you have adrenalin flowing through your blood and you are acting with full force and emotion. It is helpful to play act a bit, encourage your partner to respond realistically to your strikes. Generally we recoil, or close our body up, when we experience pain.

This will create a dynamic interaction and change your partner's body position, exposing new targets and allowing more options for you.

If you choose to practice scenarios that involve guns, knives or other sharp weapons, do not use live weapons. Accidents can easily happen. Use a replica, or something that looks like the weapon and gives you the appropriate practice. If you practice with a gun, even a toy one, the person holding the gun should not put their finger on the trigger. Fingers are is easily broken if they get tangled during a disarm.

Be aware also of other people around you as you practice these scenarios. It is best to do these in private and not make a lot of noise, or a bystander may quite rightly call law enforcement or step in to assist.

If you can, it is also helpful to attend classes or seminars on self defense techniques with a qualified instructor. They will be able to give you many further tips on how to deal with situations you may find yourself in and how to use your body effectively. They will also be able to tailor these tips to you personally, something which can not be done easily through the medium of a book.

Basic principles

Use your presence

If the attack has not already ensued, verbally address your attacker and warn them away. Assume a confident, ready posture. Look fierce. Yell and scream if your opponent continues. Refer back to chapter seven for details on this. Get into the habit now so you do it automatically when you need to.

Wallets, cellphones, handbags etc

Remember that our objective is to keep ourselves and our loved ones safe. If all our attacker wants is some kind of physical possession, just give it to them if it is safe to do so. Remember violent confrontations are unpredictable. You have prepared yourself well, but you still do not know what the outcome of a situation will be. If you can avoid violence, do it. It is not worth risking harm to ourselves, our loved ones or even our attacker for that matter over some kind of physical possession which can be replaced.

Check for escape routes

Is there a way you can get away from the attacker without using violence? If you can walk or run from the situation in a way which is safe for yourself and others around you, do so.

Attack suddenly and ferociously

You want to overwhelm your attacker with the suddenness of your attack. You want to strike quickly and repeatedly at sensitive targets putting our attacker on the back foot. Of course in a real situation not everything will always go your way, not all your strikes will connect cleanly and you may find yourself also being struck and moved around. Keeping up a constant barrage of strikes will make it more difficult for your attacker than if you remain passive. It also increases the chance of landing an effective strike which causes pain or impairment to your attacker. This then leaves your attacker open to further effective strikes and may lead to them breaking off their attack and retreating

Use your best weapons

Use any available object as a weapon. If no suitable weapons are available use the most effective parts of your body as a weapon. Refer back to chapter eight for details on this.

Grabs, chokes and pins

Often a larger stronger opponent will try to grab hold of you in some way to force you to submit to their will. Ideally we do not want this to happen. Ideally we want to strike and deal to our attacker before this happens.

If an attacker does manage to grab you, your best defense is not to worry too much about how exactly they are holding or pinning you, but just strike as ferociously as you can at whatever sensitive targets you can reach with whatever weapon you can. This will quickly take their mind off their grip or hold making it easier to break free. This is the most important thing. We will not go into specific techniques here. There are dozens of them. As long as you inflict enough pain on your attacker, breaking free will not generally be a problem.

When we do break free we go through the weakest point of the hold. For the hands this means through the thumb (one thumb is much weaker than four fingers). This works even better if you use your other hand to create a "push-pull" action.

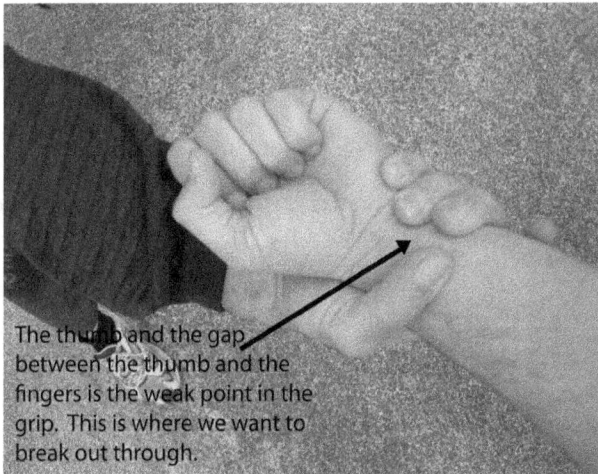

The thumb and the gap between the thumb and the fingers is the weak point in the grip. This is where we want to break out through.

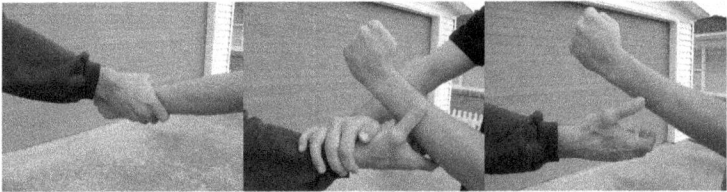

Exactly how this works will depend on the nature of the grab. Experiment and find what works for you.

For a headlock or some sort of embrace this means exiting through underneath the armpit.

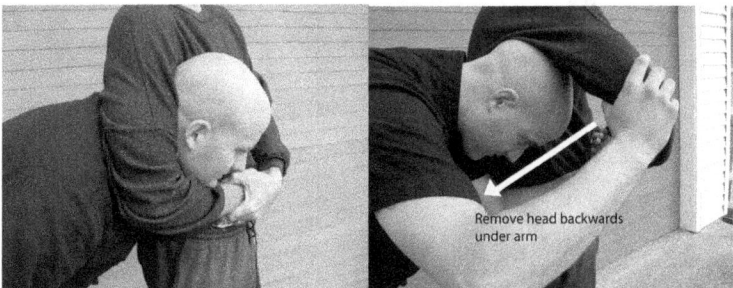

Remove head backwards under arm

Leaving the scene

As soon as you feel you are able to, leave the scene and get help. Call emergency services, let the police know what has happened and obtain medical services if they are needed for either you or your attacker.

Attackers with weapons

There are three types of weapons you are most likely to be faced with, long weapons such as bats and bars, sharp weapons such as knives and bottles, and finally guns. Dealing with these weapons can be tricky, particularly knives and guns. A slight slip can cause serious injury or death. Do not take them lightly. We will look at a few basic principles here, but remember the first option is always to avoid violence unless absolutely necessary. Only physically engage with your attacker if you think they actually intend to use the weapon they are carrying. If dealing with an attacker with weapons is a major concern of yours it would pay to attend in person training which specifically focuses on this area.

Bats and bars

The most dangerous point on this weapon is the end. As you progress up towards the attacker, the force and damage becomes less and less.

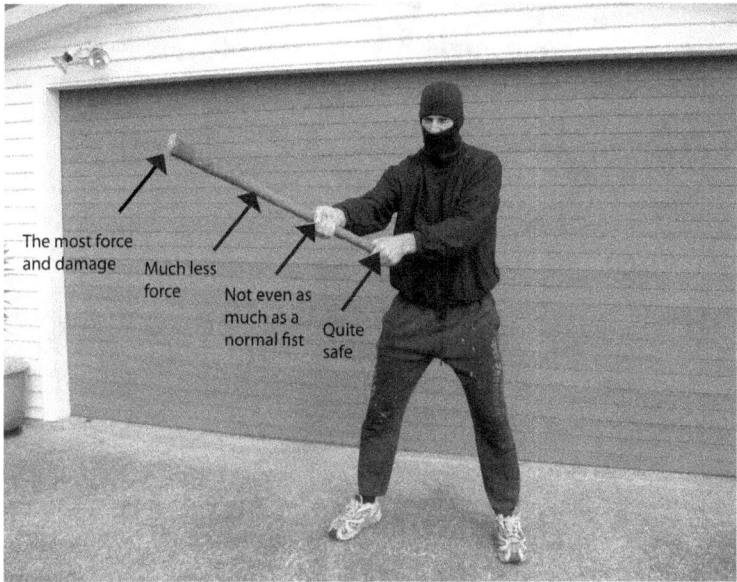

The most force and damage
Much less force
Not even as much as a normal fist
Quite safe

Commonly people will swing this type of weapon. They will generally pull the weapon backwards before they swing in with a hit. To deal with this it is best to get close to them as quickly as possible into a range where you can strike them and the weapon is no longer as effective. If they take you by surprise you may need to dodge the first swing and then close in rapidly while the weapon is still recoiled.

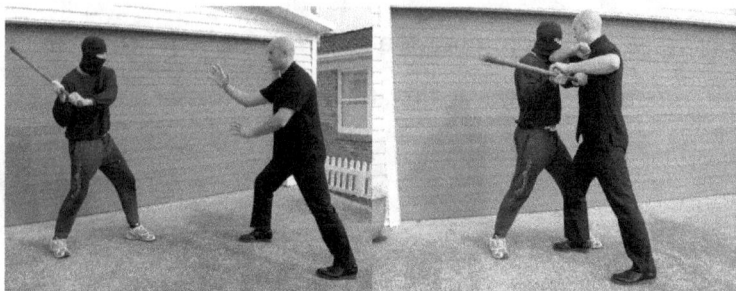

Closing in immediately will move you past the most dangerous part of
a long swinging weapon.

Knives

Knives are very versatile weapons able to twist, turn and cut
through the full range of motion of the wrist. There is a
rule of thumb that if a knife is pulled someone will get cut,
possibly both. The real question is how badly. If at all
possible you want to put something between you and the
knife. This could be furniture such as a chair, an article of
clothing, any available object to deflect the blade and tangle
it if possible.

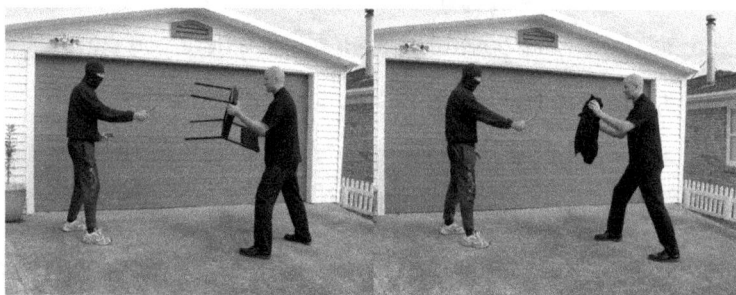

Anything you can use to intercept the knife is useful.

Another option if you are wearing shoes is to kick at the attacker. Shoes can be quite tough to cut through and any cuts to the feet and lower legs are preferable to cuts to the hands, arms, abdomen and face.

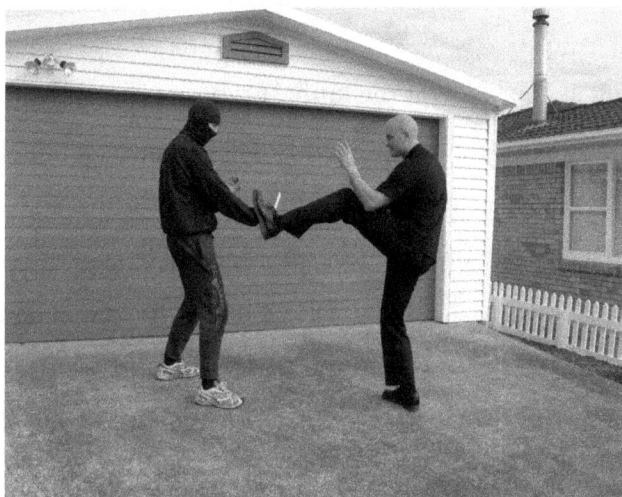

Shoes act as good protection against a blade.

If no such items are available, and you are not confident with your kicking ability, you may need to engage with your attacker hand to hand. Intercept the forearm of the knife hand with your arm to keep the blade away from your body. Immediately clamp your other hand on the knife butt end of their hand. This stops the knife from being rotated and cutting your hands and arms. The pictures below show an intercept and then clamping of the hand in the two most common knife grips.

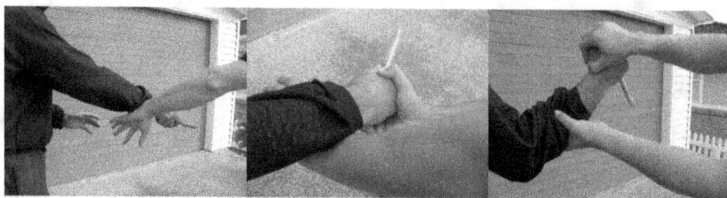

The hand is gripped on the opposing side to the blade, whichever grip the attacker is using.

As long as the blade of the knife is exposed it is still a threat to you. It can be quite difficult to safely remove a knife from an attacker's hand without extensive practice and experience. One of the safest ways for you to cover the knife's blade is with your attacker's body. Keep one hand clamped on the butt end of the knife hand and use the other to bend the elbow and drive the knife into your attacker.

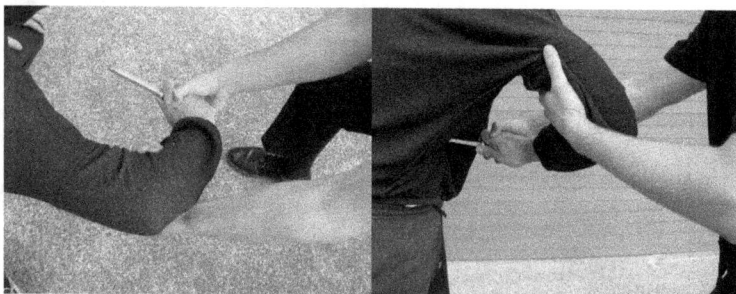

Use the other hand to fold the elbow, redirecting the blade in towards the attacker.

Guns

A gun is most effective from a distance. From a distance there is little that you can effectively do against an attacker with a gun except talk them down. If absolutely necessary you can throw something at them to distract them and then attempt to close the distance between you, or find cover. If the attacker is very close, you have the option of retrieving the gun from them. To do this, bring the hands up suddenly, deflecting the gun to the side as you move your body in the other direction. Grab the barrel of the gun and twist up then down. This will break the attackers grip on the weapon and possibly the finger on the trigger. Take the gun from their hand and step back to a safe distance with the gun trained on them.

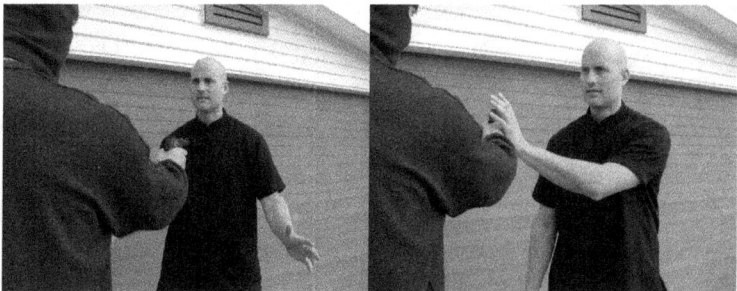

Step to the side at the same time as you push the gun to the other side. You only need to move the gun a few inches to be out of the line of fire.

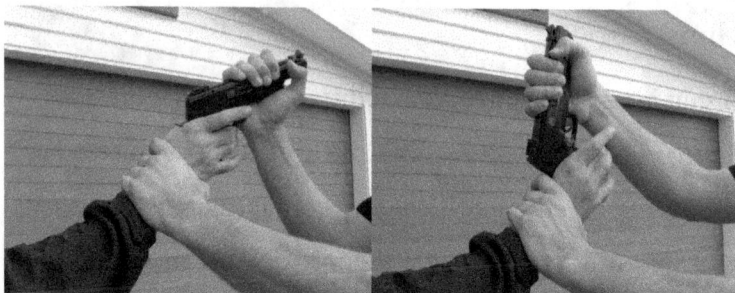

Grab the barrel and push up (when practicing make sure your partner does not have their finger inside the trigger guard).

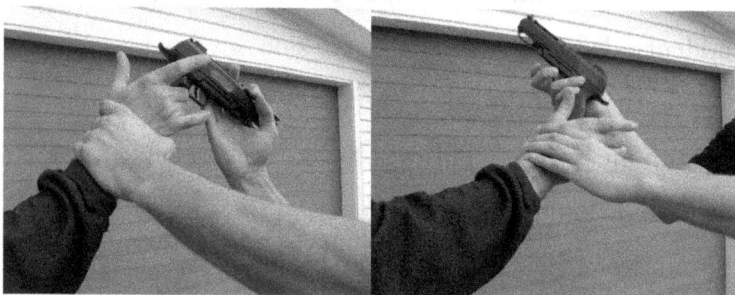

Pull the barrel back downwards, breaking the grip. Remove the gun from the attacker's hand.

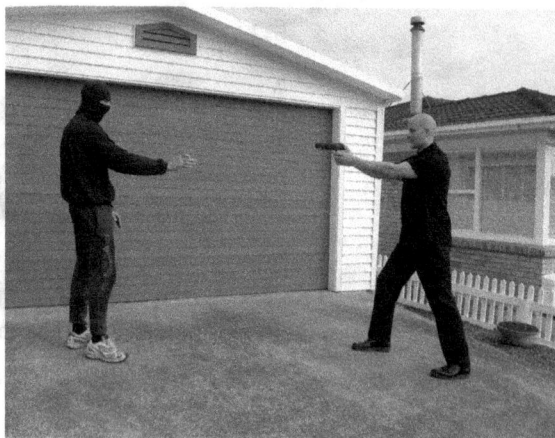

Step back away from the attacker so they can not disarm you in a similar way.

Scenarios:

In the bathroom

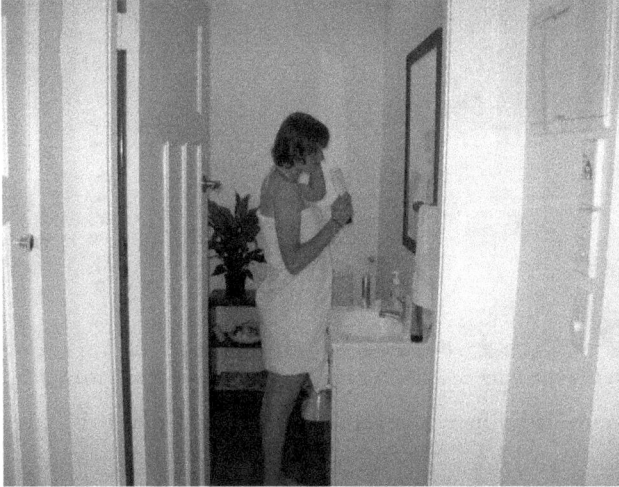

An attack can occur anywhere, even in your own bathroom. The intended victim is minding her own business brushing her hair.

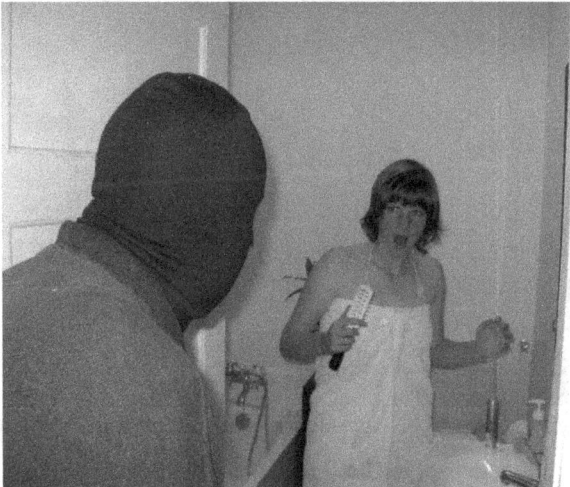

An intruder enters. The intended victim screams and yells at the intruder.

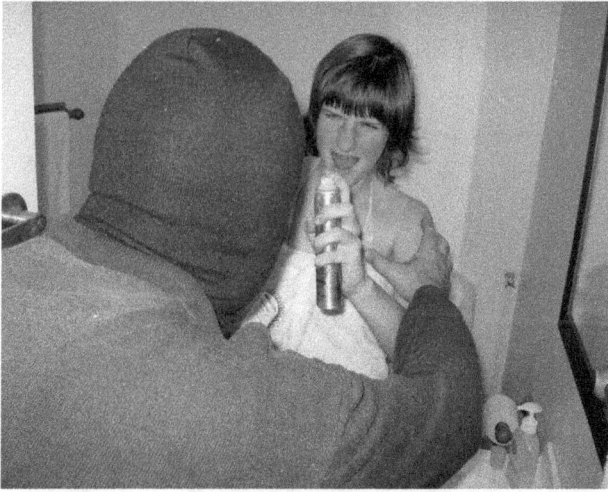

When the intruder reaches for her it is clear he intends to attack. She immediately sprays the aerosol can she has handy in his face.

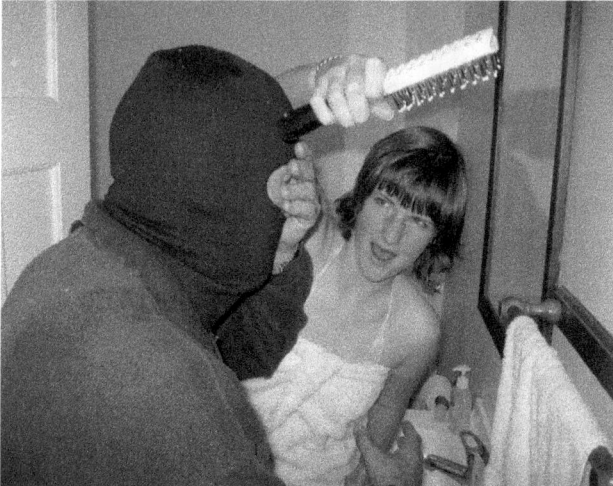

She then strikes the attacker repeatedly in the temple and face with the handle of the hairbrush she is holding.

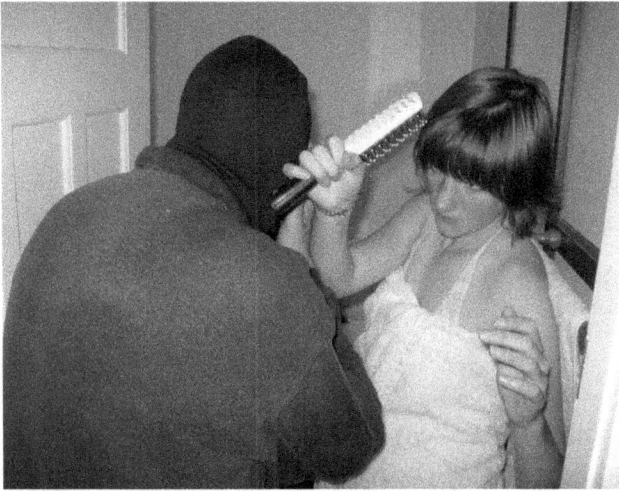

She continues to strike around the clavicle and neck as the attacker covers his face with his hands.

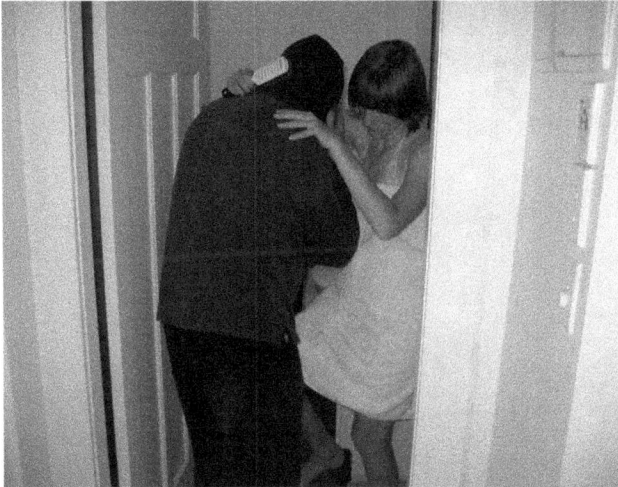

She then knees the attacker in the groin causing him to bend forwards.

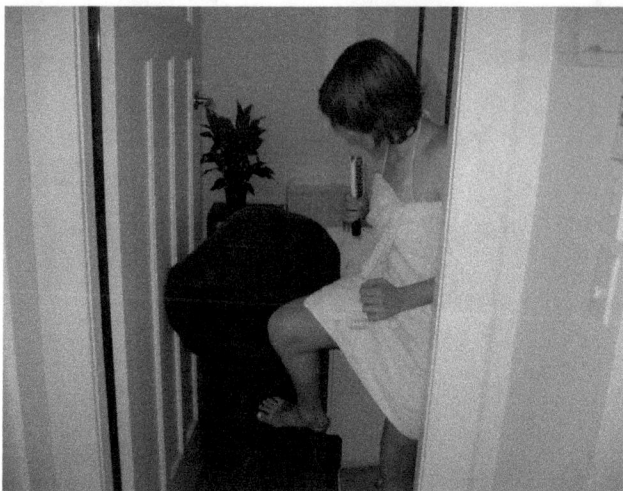
As the attacker stumbles she stomps on the back of his knee.

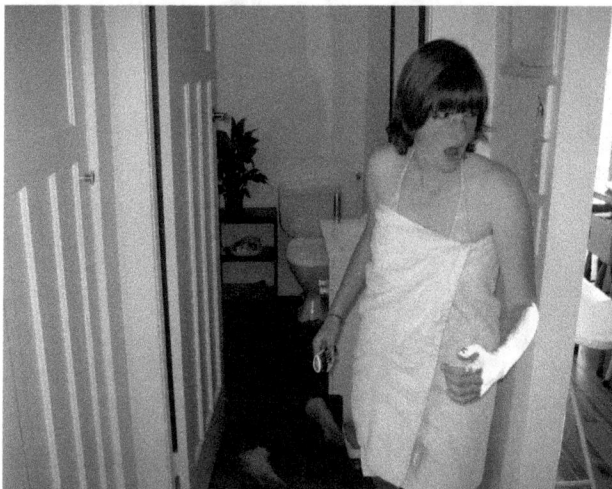
This sends the attacker to the ground. She is now free to make her escape…

Running through a park

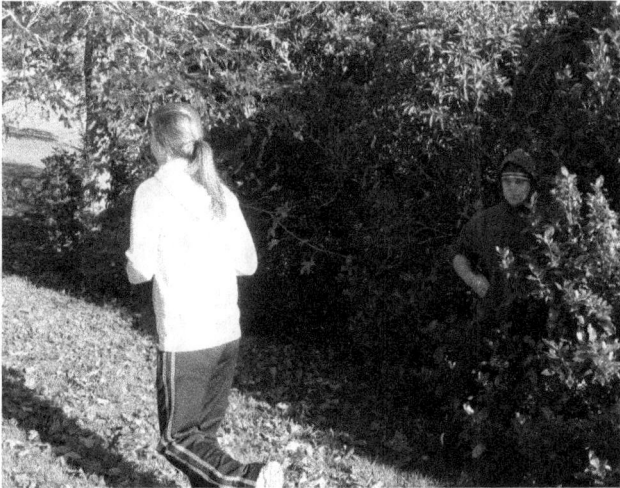
The intended victim is jogging through a park

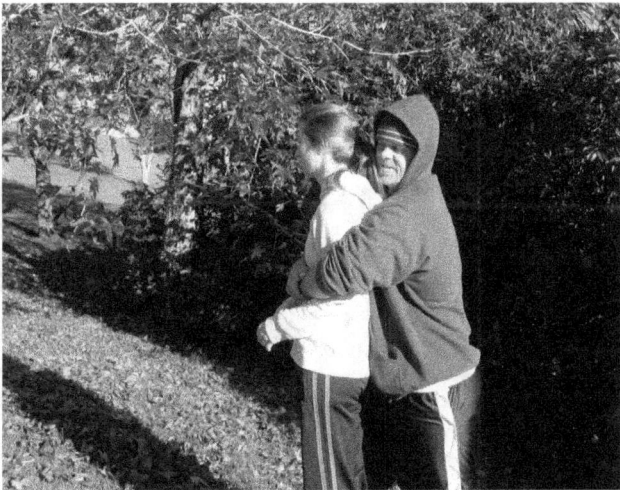
An attacker jumps out from behind some bushes, putting her in a bear hug trapping both her arms

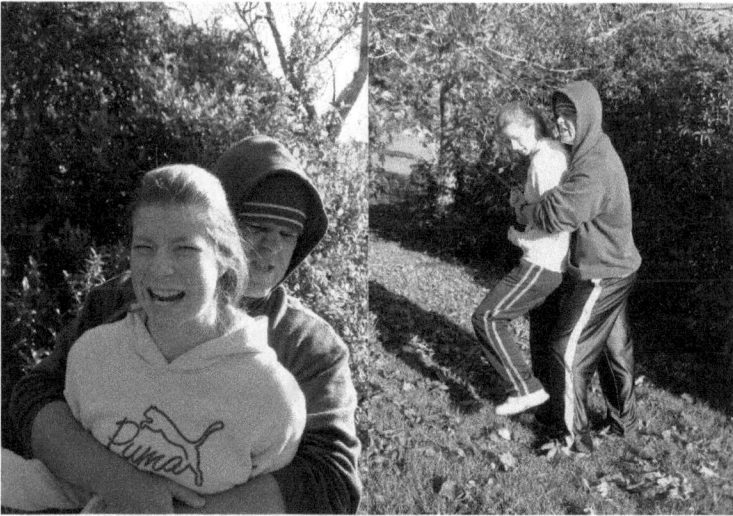

She immediately screams for help and then suddenly stomps down
hard on the attacker's foot with her heel.

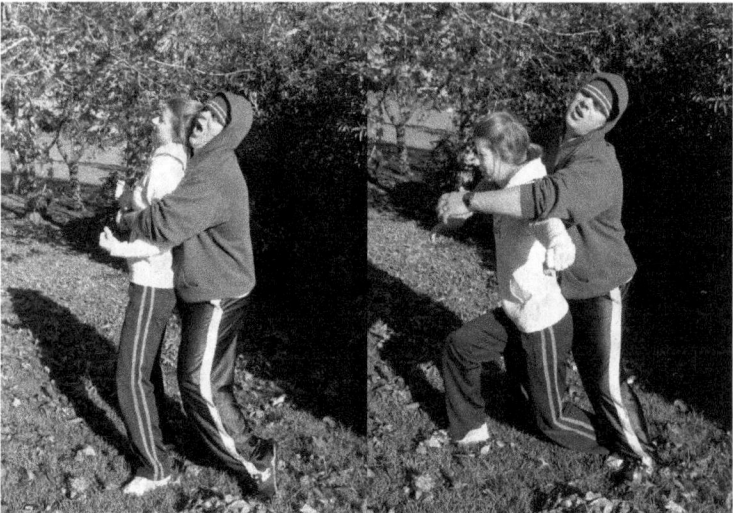

She follows this straight away with a head butt backwards to loosen the
attacker's grip. She breaks free by dropping her weight downwards and
pushing both her arms out hard to the side.

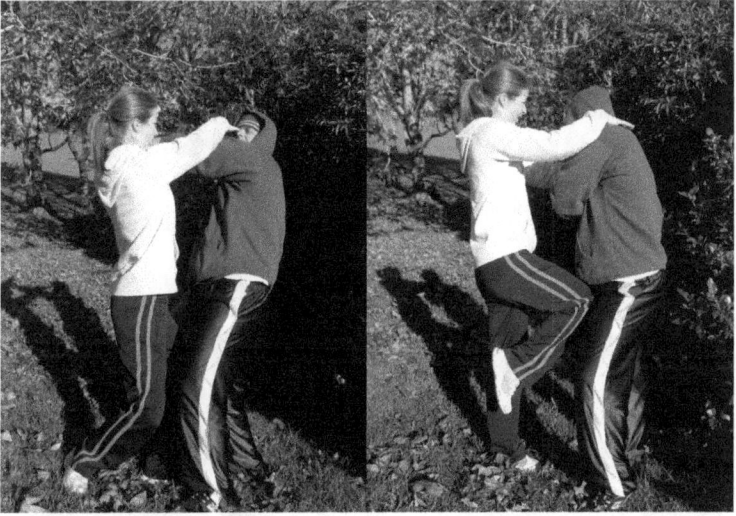

She clears the attacker's arms and thrusts her fingers into his eyes, following this with a knee to the groin.

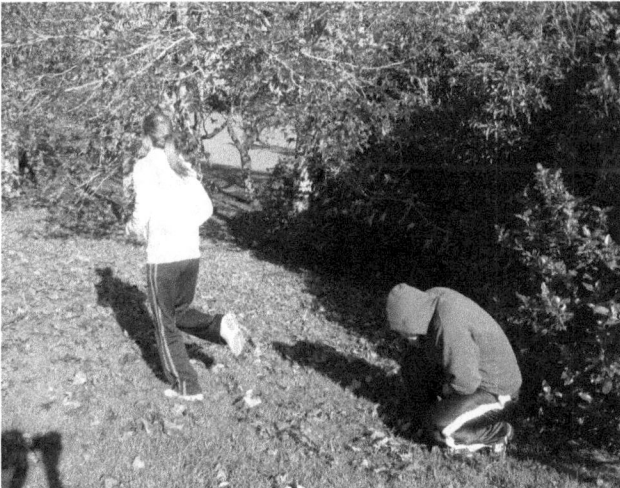

As soon as she is able, she runs from her attacker, continuing to yell for assistance as she goes.

Getting into your car

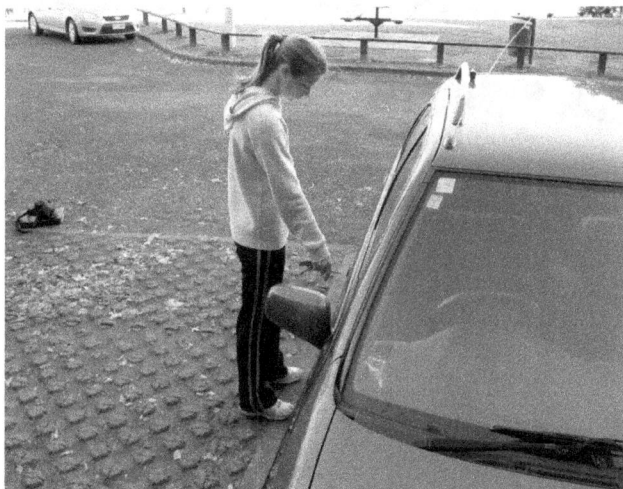

The intended victim is unlocking her car.

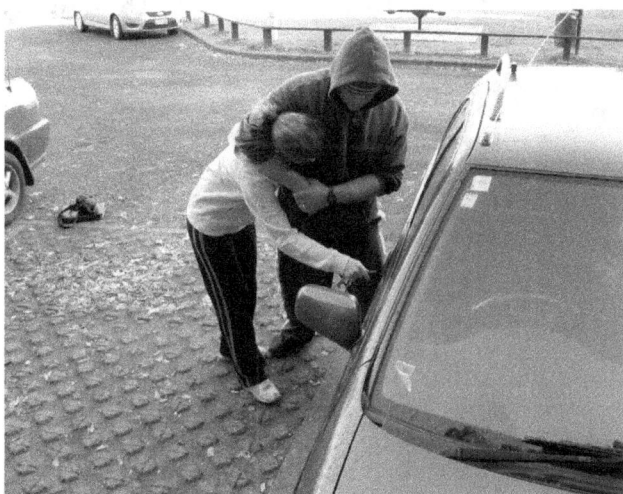

An attacker comes on her from behind, putting her in a head lock.

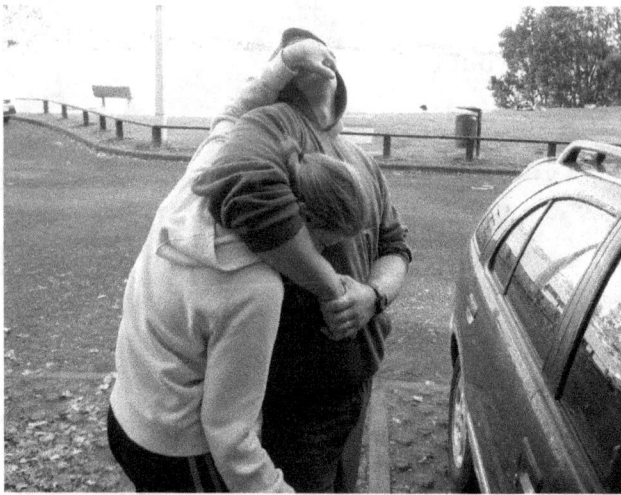

She screams and immediately reaches her hand around behind her attacker's head and pushes backwards with her fingers gouging the face and eyes.

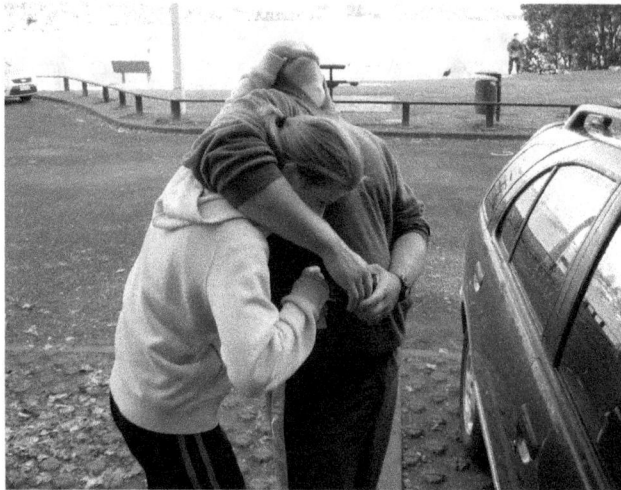

She then thrusts the key she has in her hand into her attacker's ribs.

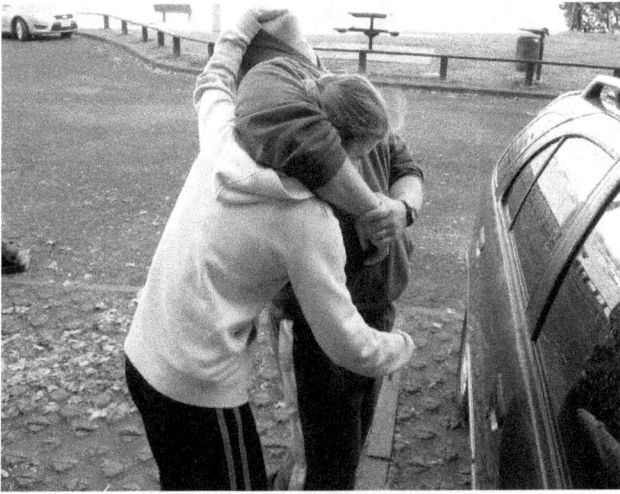

She follows this with strikes to the groin.

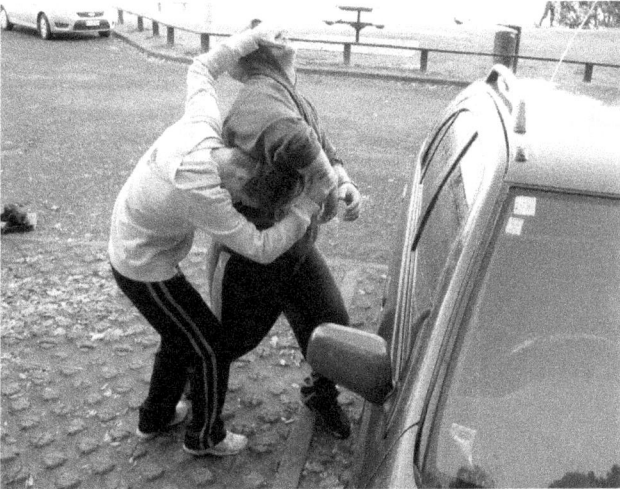

She now pushes free of her attacker, coming out from under his arm.

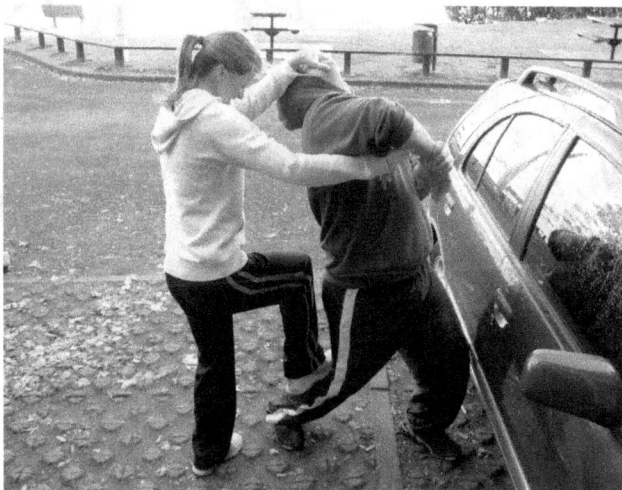

She stomps down hard on the back of her attacker's knee, bringing him to the ground.

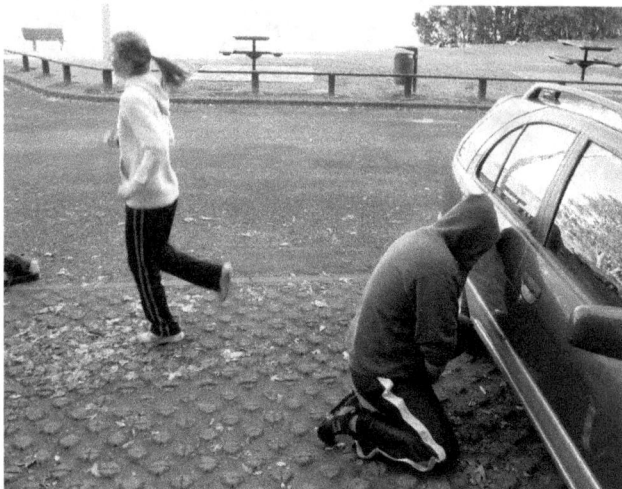

She now takes her opportunity to run from the situation, calling for assistance as she goes.

In the bedroom

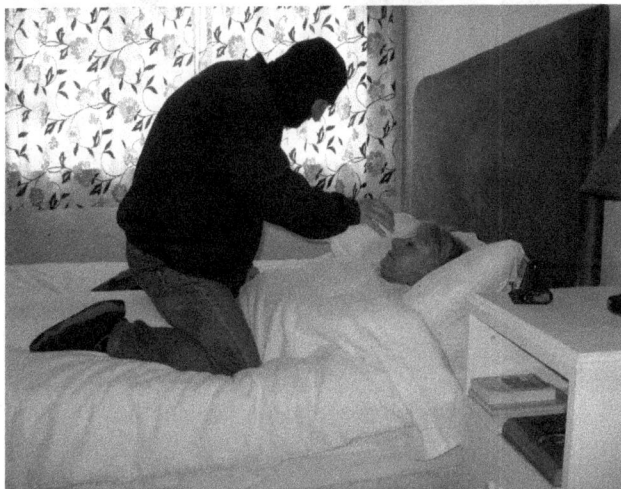

The intended victim wakes up with and intruder on top of her.

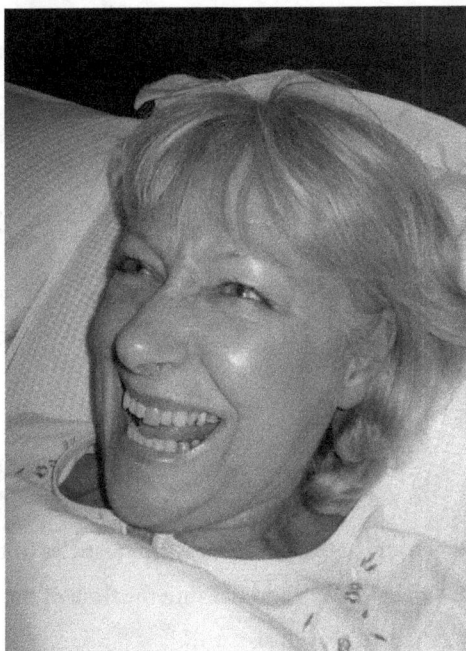

She immediately screams for help.

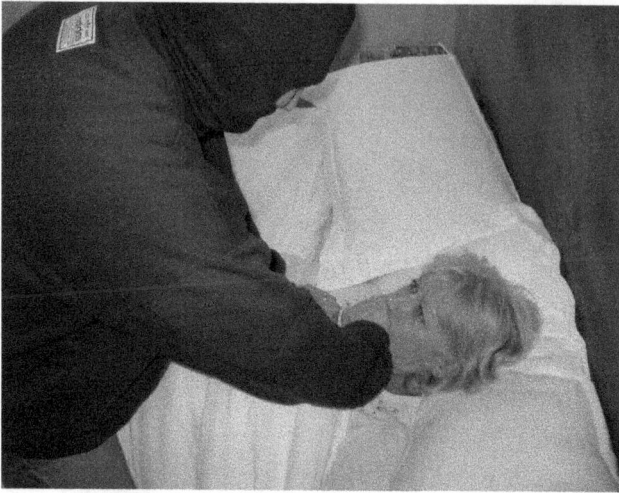

The attacker goes to cover her mouth.

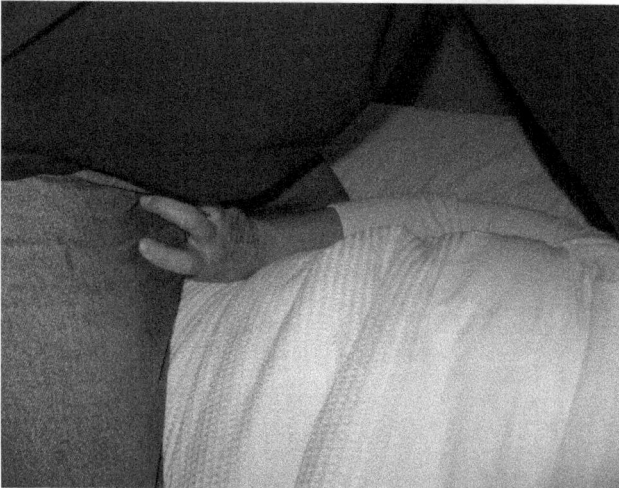

She reaches down and grabs and squeezes his testicles (if the testicles can't be reached the grabbing and twisting the flesh of the inner thigh will also work).

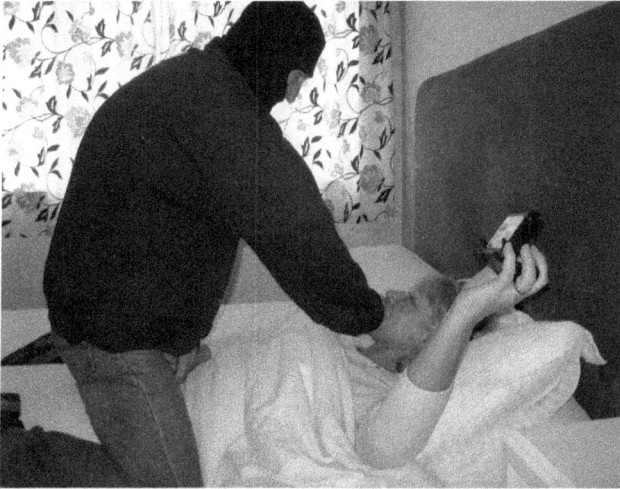

The grab to the groin distracts him and causes him to shift his weight, making it easier to grab the alarm clock on the bedside table and…

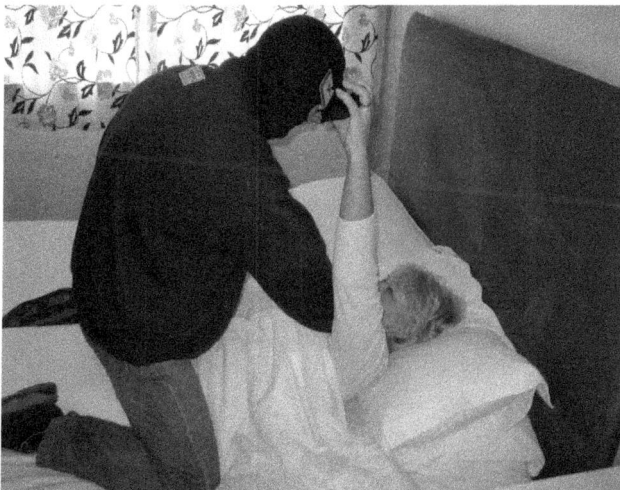

Smash the clock into the side of his head or face.

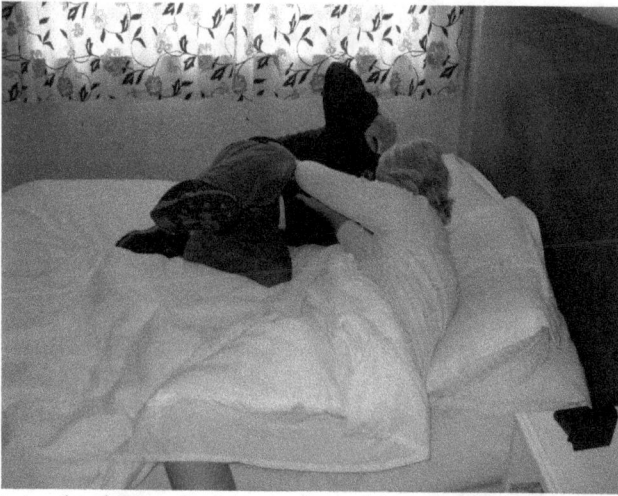

Twisting her hips and pushing, she is able to get out from under her attacker

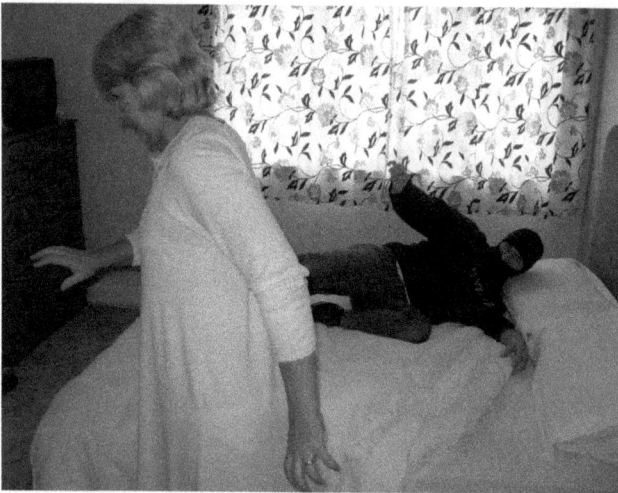

And run from the room, calling for help as she goes.

In the street

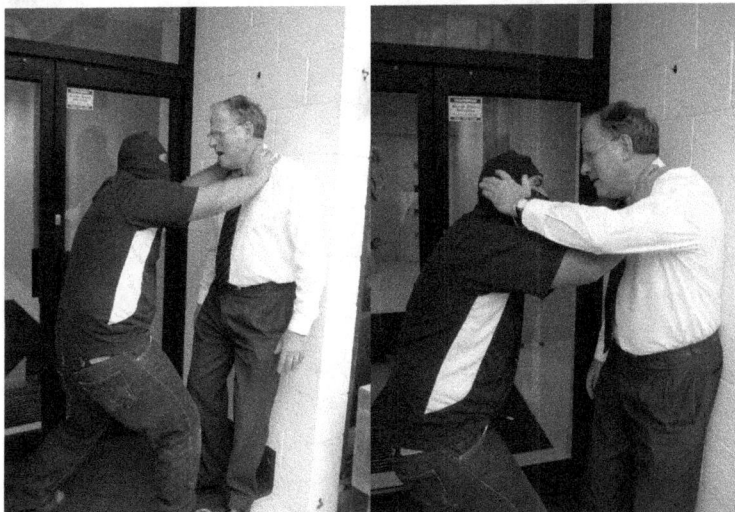

Entering a building, the intended victim is choked up against a wall.
He responds by immediately cupping his attacker across the ear.

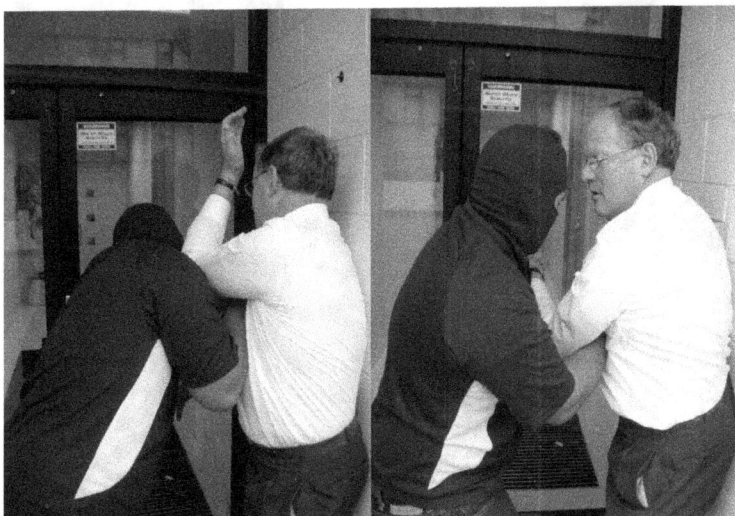

He brings his elbow over and down to free his attackers hands from his
neck.

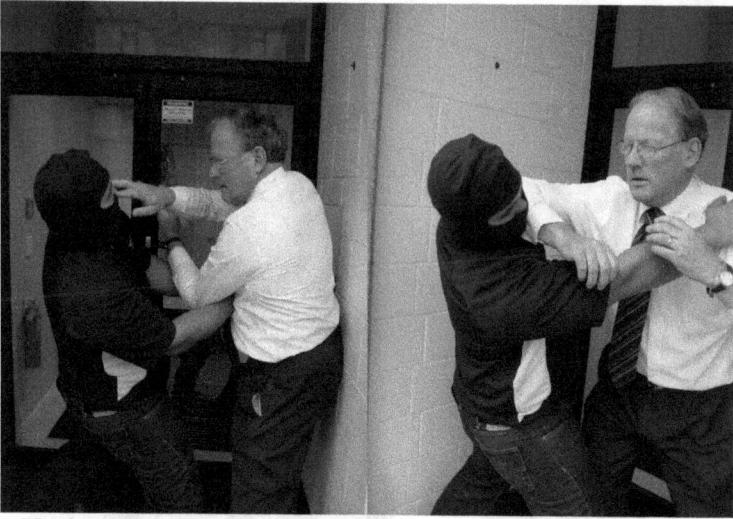

He then immediately strikes the attacker in the eyes, followed by an elbow to the jaw.

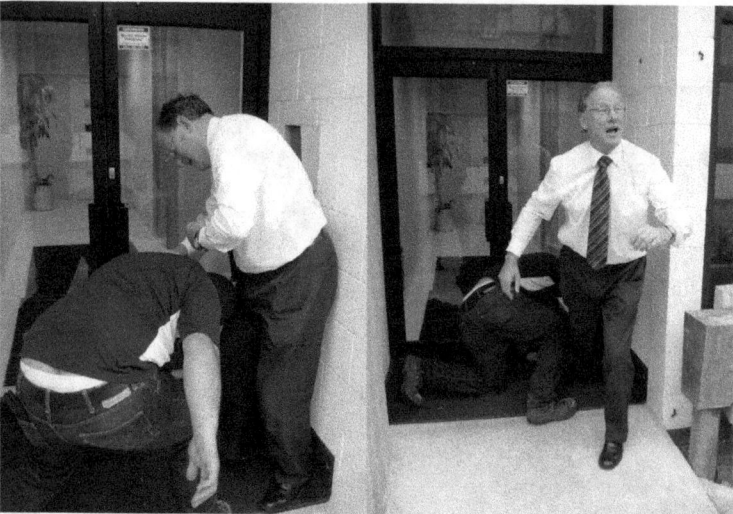

He then pulls his attacker down, striking him in the back of the neck with a hammer fist before escaping from the scene, calling for help as he goes.

In the kitchen

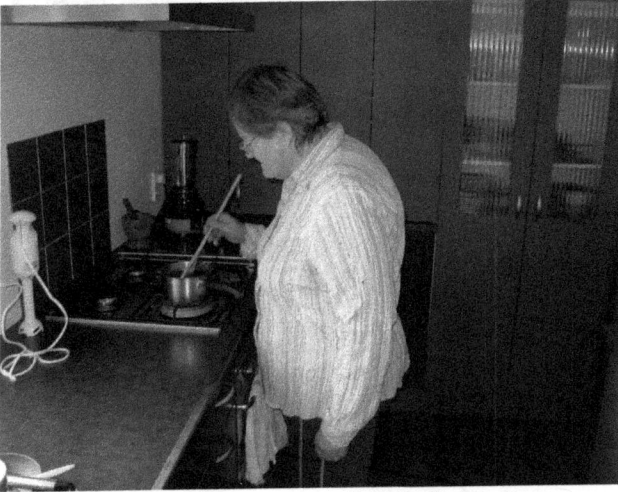

The intended victim is cooking in the kitchen.

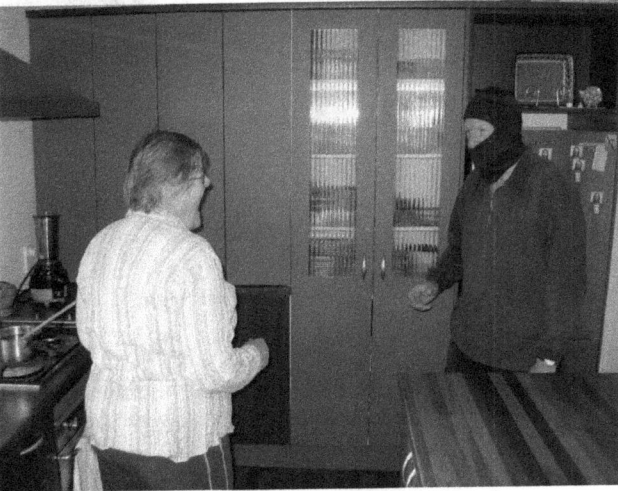

She hears an intruder, turns and yells at him.

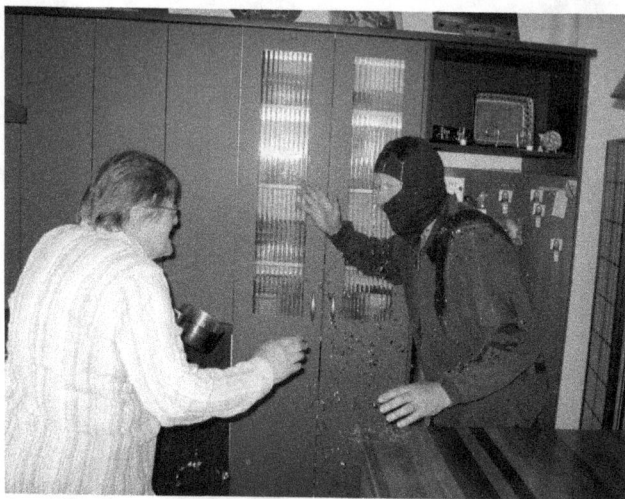

The intruder continues to advance, so she throws the hot contents of the pot on the stove at him.

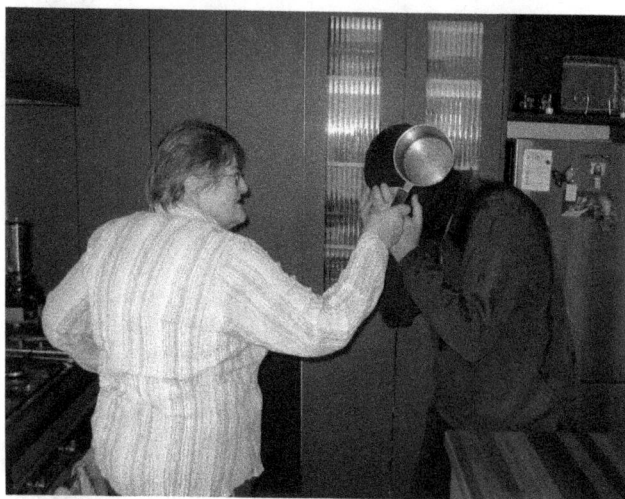

Following up by hitting him in the head with the pot.

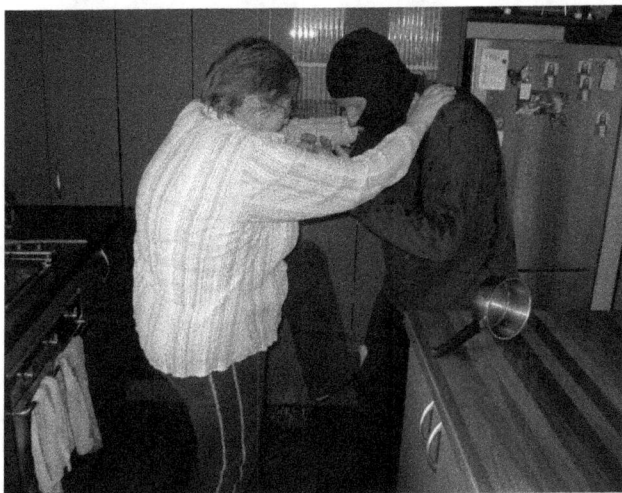

She then kicks him in the front of the knee, bringing him down and forwards.

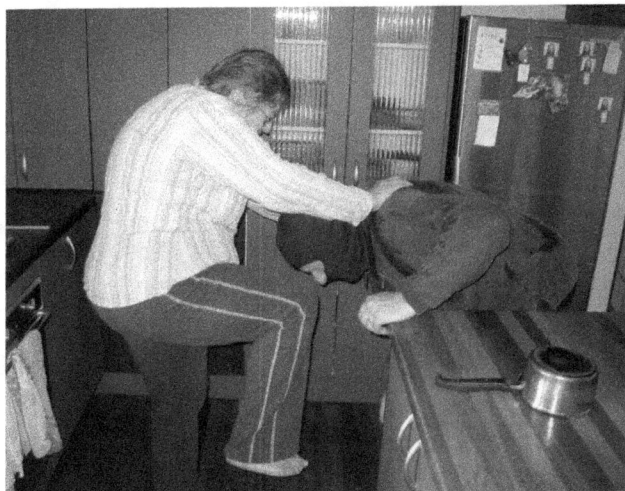

She knees him in the face as he comes forwards.

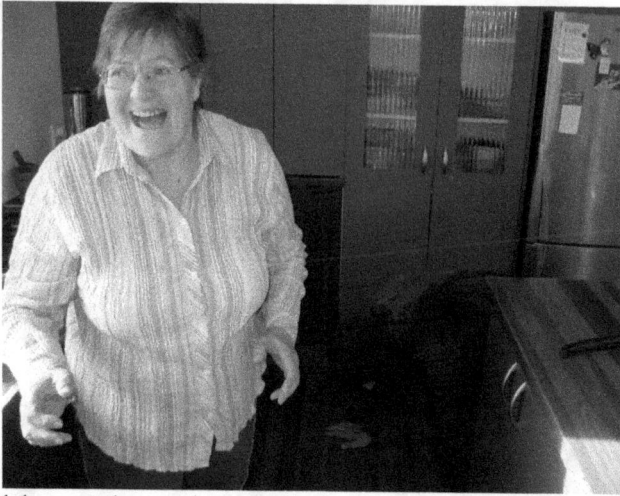
With her attacker on the ground, she now feels safe to flee the scene,
calling for assistance as she goes.

In the Office

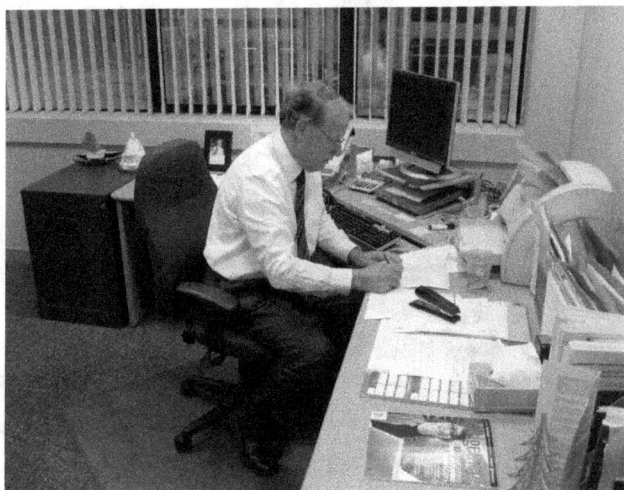

In the office.

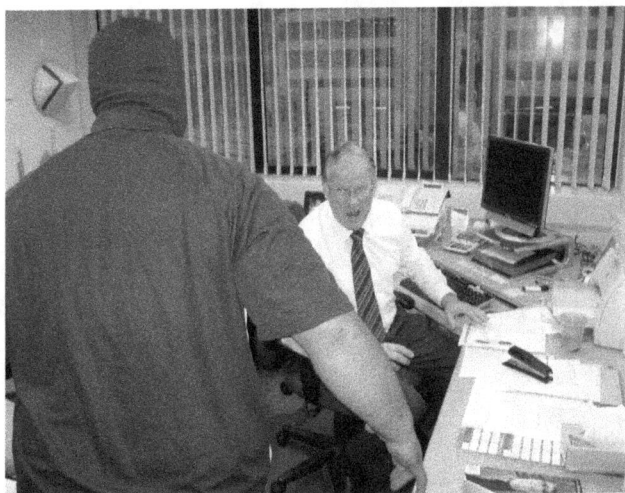

An intruder enters. The intended victim immediately yells at the intruder.

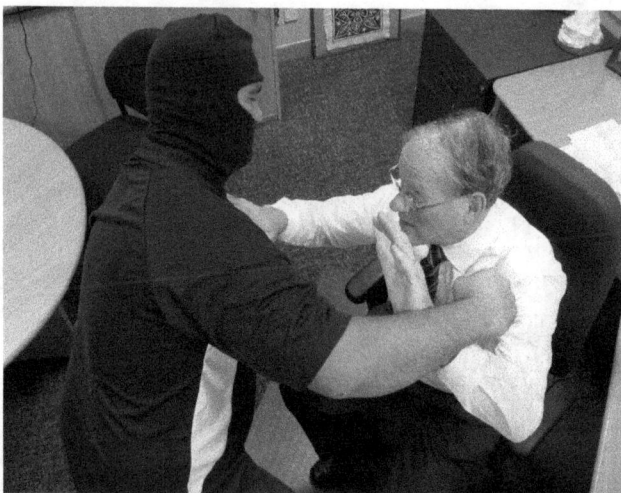

The intruder throws a punch at the intended victim. There is no time to pick up a weapon, so he covers up with one hand – taking the punch on his arm. The other hand simultaneously jabs fingers first into the base of the attacker's throat.

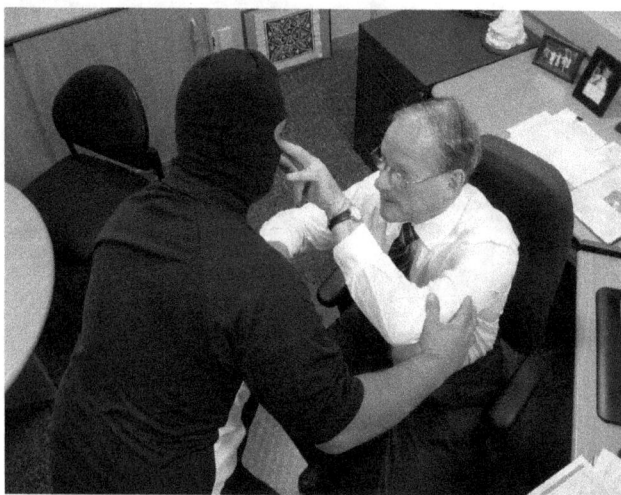

Followed straight away by a finger jab to the eyes.

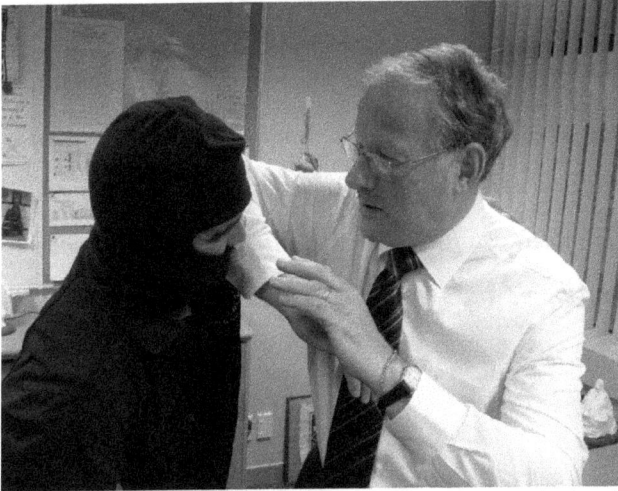

He the stands up into his attacker, elbowing him in the head.

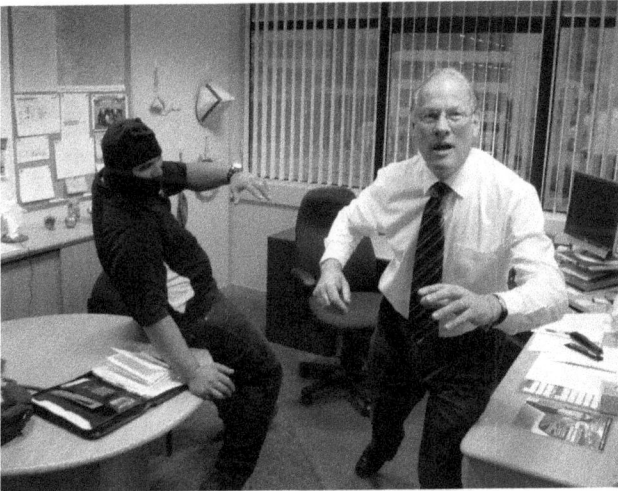

This knocks the attacker backwards giving a chance to escape, yelling for help as he goes.

Exercise 8:

Find a partner you trust who you can practice scenarios such as these with. Make the scenarios as realistic as possible while still being safe. Experiment with different ways of dealing with the situation until you find ones that suit you. Practice until you are comfortable and confident.

Chapter Eleven: A picture of contentedness

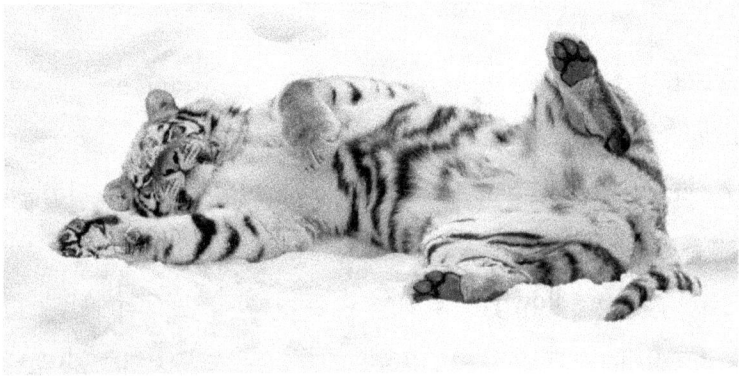

Cats are wonderful animals, graceful and independent. Most of the time they are relaxed and calm, happy exploring a new nook, playing and hunting, or just stretching out taking a nap in the sun.

In this book we have covered some extremely violent and quite graphic material. For some of us this may have been quite distasteful. As has been mentioned several times, this kind of violence is to be avoided if at all possible. However the reality of our modern society is that many of us will have cause to use what we have learned in this book at one time or another.

We can learn a lot from the cat in our story. The cat doesn't go around tense and worried about being attacked.

Far from it. Most of the time the cat is the very picture of relaxation and enjoyment; only using the violent skills we have looked at in this book when it really needs to.

When it does need to, it transforms in an instant, acting almost faster than we can see. The speed of this transformation and action is due in part to how relaxed the cat was in the first place. You see, when we are tense, we respond more slowly. Tension means we are either still responding to something in the past, or we are responding to something in the future which has not happened yet, or we are responding internally to a current situation with fear but not acting externally in response to that situation fully effectively. Inside we are fighting ourselves. We are using that tension to hold our selves in a particular position which is not useful to us, whether that position is psychological or physical. When the situation changes and we are faced with new circumstances, our reactions are slowed because we first have to overcome the existing tension.

When we regularly go about our daily activities in a state of tension, we are wasting energy. We are habitually releasing small amounts of adrenalin into our bloodstream to maintain the tension. When the time comes that we really need our body to respond to the release of adrenalin, it will take more of it to achieve the same effect a smaller amount would have previously had as our bodies have become habituated to the presence of adrenalin in our system, much as it does to any chemical. Also our ability to release adrenalin will be reduced. Our adrenal glands will have become tired and weakened from constantly having to produce and release adrenalin without a break to rest and restore themselves.

It is in our best interests to be as relaxed as we can throughout most of our daily lives.

The cat with a tiger inside is so relaxed because it is prepared. It knows the realities of what it might face and has prepared itself for them. In the mean time it just gets on with enjoying its life, alert, but relaxed.

We can do the same. By facing the realities of what is necessary to protect ourselves and by completing the exercises contained in this book we can prepare ourselves to deal with the situations we might face. We can then more easily get on with our lives, alert, but relaxed, confident that when the time comes we will be able to let out THE TIGER WITHIN.

Checklists

Always:

1. **Stake out your environment.** Know where threats may come from; know where safe havens and escape routes are.
2. **Remain Alert.** Put yourself in a position where you can be forewarned of danger. Raise your head from what you are doing periodically.
3. **Identify possible threats.** Pay attention to the people around you. Learn to recognize the signals they send.
4. **Use your presence.** Have confident posture. Verbally address any potential threat. Scream and yell if necessary.
5. **Practice likely scenarios.** Play through likely scenarios both mentally and physically to prepare yourself to act quickly, confidently and decisively.
6. **Relax.** Make whatever preparations you need to and then relax. You will respond better from a relaxed, comfortable state than from one of worry and fear.

In case of violence:

1. **Use your presence.** Assume a ferocious look. Yell and scream at your attacker and for help.

2. **If your attacker wants money or some other physical possession – just give it to them.**

3. **Check for escape routes.** If there is a safe way for you to leave the situation without violence, do so.

4. **Use your best weapons.** These may be items you are carrying or something you can pick up and use, or they may be parts of your body.

5. **Attack the most sensitive targets on your opponent's body.** Maximize your effectiveness by striking the areas of your opponent's body most susceptible to pain and damage.

6. **Attack ferociously.** Strike repetitively at your opponent overwhelming their senses.

7. **Break out of grabs or holds through the weakest point.** This means through the gap between the thumb and the fingers, or under the armpit.

8. **Leave the scene.** As soon as possible leave the area, get help and alert the authorities.

About the author

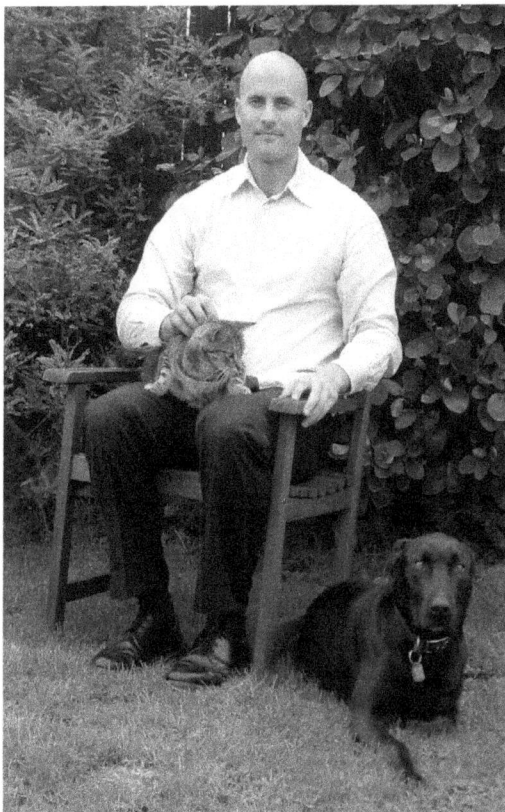

John lives in Auckland, New Zealand with his cat George AND his dog Jenny. There he practices Traditional Chinese Medicine and teaches qigong, kung fu and self defense. The style of kung fu he practices is the Wah family southern tiger style. His qualifications include: Diploma Traditional Chinese Medicine, Diploma Qigong, Certified Neuro Linguistic Programming practitioner, Registered Personal Trainer.

He can be reached via his website at: www.developyourqi.com

120